PAIN AND ITS ORIGINS, DIAGNOSIS AND TREATMENTS

PHARMACOLOGICAL INTERVENTION IN MANAGEMENT OF NECK PAIN DISORDERS: A REVIEW

PAIN AND ITS ORIGINS, DIAGNOSIS AND TREATMENTS

Additional books in this series can be found on Nova's website under the Series tab.

Additional E-books in this series can be found on Nova's website under the E-books tab.

PAIN AND ITS ORIGINS, DIAGNOSIS AND TREATMENTS

PHARMACOLOGICAL INTERVENTION IN MANAGEMENT OF NECK PAIN DISORDERS: A REVIEW

MARWAN S.M. AL-NIMER

Nova Biomedical
Nova Science Publishers, Inc.
New York

Copyright © 2010 by Nova Science Publishers, Inc.

All rights reserved. No part of this book may be reproduced, stored in a retrieval system or transmitted in any form or by any means: electronic, electrostatic, magnetic, tape, mechanical photocopying, recording or otherwise without the written permission of the Publisher.

For permission to use material from this book please contact us:
Telephone 631-231-7269; Fax 631-231-8175
Web Site: http://www.novapublishers.com

NOTICE TO THE READER
The Publisher has taken reasonable care in the preparation of this book, but makes no expressed or implied warranty of any kind and assumes no responsibility for any errors or omissions. No liability is assumed for incidental or consequential damages in connection with or arising out of information contained in this book. The Publisher shall not be liable for any special, consequential, or exemplary damages resulting, in whole or in part, from the readers' use of, or reliance upon, this material.

Independent verification should be sought for any data, advice or recommendations contained in this book. In addition, no responsibility is assumed by the publisher for any injury and/or damage to persons or property arising from any methods, products, instructions, ideas or otherwise contained in this publication.

This publication is designed to provide accurate and authoritative information with regard to the subject matter covered herein. It is sold with the clear understanding that the Publisher is not engaged in rendering legal or any other professional services. If legal or any other expert assistance is required, the services of a competent person should be sought. FROM A DECLARATION OF PARTICIPANTS JOINTLY ADOPTED BY A COMMITTEE OF THE AMERICAN BAR ASSOCIATION AND A COMMITTEE OF PUBLISHERS.

Library of Congress Cataloging-in-Publication Data
Al-Nimer, Marwan S. M.
  Pharmacological intervention in management of neck pain disorders : a review / Marwan S.M. Al-Nimer.
    p. ; cm.
  Includes bibliographical references and index.
  ISBN 978-1-61728-221-8 (softcover)
  1. Neck pain--Chemotherapy. I. Title.
  [DNLM: 1. Neck Pain--drug therapy. 2. Analgesics--therapeutic use. 3. Neck Pain--etiology. WE 708 A452p 2010]
  RC936.P43 2010
   615'.783--dc22
                                                            2010025682

Published by Nova Science Publishers, Inc. ✝ *New York*

Contents

Preface		vii
Chapter I	Introduction	1
Chapter II	Pain Perception	3
Chapter III	Central, Topical and Peripherally Acting Analgesics	17
Chapter IV	Antimicrobials	49
Chapter V	Complementary/Alternative Analgesia	55
Chapter VI	Quality of Life	71
Conclusion		75
References		77
Index		115

Preface

The prevalence of neck pain disorders is increasing worldwide. Approximately 10% of adult have neck pain at any one time and less than 1% develop neurological deficit. The treatment of neck pain depends on its precise cause. It includes: rest, heat/ice application, traction, soft collar traction, physical therapy, transcutaneous electric nerve stimulation, surgical procedures and pharmacotherapy. The current pharmacological agents that used in management of neck pain include: non steroidal anti-inflammatory drugs, centrally acting analgesia, acetaminophen, muscle relaxants, topical painkillers and/or topical anesthesia, local steroids and/or local anesthetics injections and antimicrobials. This review focuses on the concepts of pharmacotherapy of neck pain disorders in respect to the cause of neck pain, the nature of pain (acute, chronic, neuropathic or nociceptive), the mechanism of drug action, the practice of local injections with radiologist intervention, quality of life and the long term harmful effects including medicines abused. Also this review describes the beneficial effect of tumor necrosis factor-alpha (TNF-α) blockers, calcitonin gene related peptide antagonists, antimicrobials particularly in infectious cervical discitis and the traditional medicines including natural plants and herbs.

Chapter I

Introduction

Cervical spine controls the head movement, therefore, a person's ability to direct his or her organs of sensation. When bone, muscles, or nerves of the neck region are damaged, activities ranged from sedentary to record-setting are disrupted. Approximately 10% of adults have neck pain at any one time. Neck pain is a highly prevalent condition among the general population. Data from cross-sectional studies show that point estimates range from 10% to 35% [Makela et al., 1991; Andersson et al., 1993; Côté et al., 1998]. The incidence rates increase with age up to 40 to 60 years, and then decrease slightly [Fejer et al., 2006; Bot et al., 2004]. Neck pain is generally more common in women than in men [Fejer et al., 2006; Bot et al., 2005]. Approximately 30% of people with neck pain face restrictions in their activities of daily living [Picavet and Schouten, 2003]. The prevalence of neck pain and disability is increased in individuals with a life time history of neck injury who are involved in a motor vehicle collision [Côté et al., 2000]. There are several possible causes of neck pain, although it is often difficult to know with certainty what is causing pain (Box 1).

This is because the examination, and even imaging tests, are not able easily differentiating among the various causes. It is often not necessary to determine the cause of a person's neck pain, especially if the pain is mild. In most cases, neck pain can be treated conservatively with Over-The-Counter (OCT) pain medications, ice, heat and massage and stretching exercise at home. Co-morbidities are frequently associated with disabling neck pain including headache, low back pain, cardiovascular events and gastrointestinal problems. The incidence of widespread pain disorders increases after cervical spinal injury. In a study of 161 cases of traumatic injury, fibromyalgia syndrome was 13 times more frequent after neck injury than after lower extremity injury [Buskila et al., 1997].

Box 1. Causes of neck pain

Cervical strain
Cervical spondylosis
Cervical discogenic pain
Cervical facet syndrome
Whiplash injury
Cervical myofascial pain
Diffuse skeletal hyperostosis
Cervical spondylotic myelopathy
Cervical radiculopathy
Cervical herniated disc
Cervical osteoarthritis
Cervicogenic headache
Infection or osteomyelitis
Inflammatory rheumatologic disease
Vascular abnormality of cervical structures
Tumor or malignancy of cervical spine
Referred pain from cardiothoracic surgery
Psychogenic pain disorders
Malingering

Chapter II

Pain Perception

The definition of pain recommended by the International Association for the Study of Pain is that; it is an unpleasant sensory and emotional experience associated with actual or potential tissue damage [Merskey and Watson, 1979]. Allodynia is referred to pain in response to normally innocuous stimuli and if the intensity pain response is heightened, then it called hyperalgesia. Notiception is the detection of tissue damage by specialized receptors of Aδ and C nerve fibers. Acetylsalicylic acid and nonsteroidal anti-inflammatory drugs produce pain relief mainly by the restoration of nociceptive sensitivity to its resting state local and regional anaesthesia can prevent nociception from becoming pain. Pain due to nerve injury does not respond to analgesics such as morphine as efficiently as pain caused by tissue damage, indicating the complex relation between injury and pain.

Acute *vs* Chronic Pain

Acute neck pain is abrupt, intense pain that subsides after a period of days or weeks. It can also radiate to the head, shoulder, arms or hands. It typically resolves with rest, exercise, and other self-care measures. When it occurs, it is initially associated with specific autonomic and somatic reflexes, but these disappear in patients with chronic pain. It often relates to soft tissue injury (sprains of muscles, tendons, ligaments) or occurs suddenly and usually heals with several days or weeks. Its severity related directly to the extent of tissue injury and resolves overtime. Most people with acute neck pain respond rapidly to treatment and 90% are symptom free within 1-2 weeks. Recurrences of neck pain are common.

Chronic pain, such as low back pain, post herpetic neuralgia, fibromyalgia, are commonly triggered by an injury or disease, but may precipitated by factors other than the cause of pain. It is not the duration of pain that distinguish acute from chronic pain but, more importantly, the inability of the body to restore its physiological functions to normal homeostatic level. The intensity of the pain is out of proportion to the original injury or tissue damage. The intensity frequently bears little or no relation to the extent of tissue injury of other quantifiable pathology. All types of chronic pain lead people to seek health care but they are often not treated effectively. Chronic neck pain persists (lasts more than three months) and its source may be hard to determine. It continues despite treatment and inappropriate treatment of chronic pain runs as high as 50% [Sherman et al., 2006]. Chronic pain is common and represents a significant proportion of office visit complaints. Approximately 35% of the American population suffers from chronic pain and that is on the rise population ages [Sherman et al., 2006].

According to the nature of pain, it could be:

1. Nociceptive (inflammatory) pain. It is either somatic or visceral resulted from the consequence of trauma to peripheral tissue e.g. surgical incision, burn etc. Nociceptive neurons become hyperexcitable leading to central sensitization and thus greater perception of pain in the higher centers. It may involve the abnormal pain state of allodynia or hyperalgesia that resulted from both peripheral and central hypersensitivity.
2. Neuropathic pain. It resulted from primary lesion or dysfunction in the nervous tissue e.g. nerve trans-section. It characterized by spontaneous pain, hyperalgesia and allodynia which can persist after the initial injury is resolved [Woolf and Mannion, 1999].
3. Psychogenic pain

According to the localization, the pain could be:

1. Localized neck pain generally points to muscle strains, ligament sprains and degenerative facet or disc processes.
2. Radiated neck pain that radiates into the upper limbs frequently stems from nerve involvement.

Mediators of Pain Perception

Some chemical mediators are produced at spinal level or released locally following tissue injury or inflammation. These mediators are involved in the perception of pain via direct activation of sensory nerve endings (e.g. proton, ATP, glutamate, 5-hydroxytryptamine, histamine and bradykinin) or indirectly through sensitization of the nerve ending to the action of other stimuli (e.g. prostaglandins and cytokines such as IL-1β, IL-2, IL-6, IL-8, TNF-α.). Sometimes these mediators express regulatory effect on the sensory neurons, adjacent inflammatory cells and sympathetic nerves e.g. bradykinin, tachykinins and nerve growth factors.

Central Mediators

The dorsal horn of the spinal cord contains many transmitters and receptors that involve in the spinal mechanism of perception. Examples of these transmitters are peptides (substance P, calcitonin gene related peptide (CGRP), somatostatin, neuropeptide Y, and galanin), inhibitory amino acids (gamma aminobutyric acid (GABA), glycine), excitatory amino acids (glutamate, aspartate), nitric oxide, arachidonic acid metabolites, adenosine, endogenous opioids, endogenous cannibinoids).

Peripheral Mediators

When the nociceptors in peripheral tissues are stimulated, the nociception pulses are transmitted to the central nervous system by two types of neurons; Aδ nerve fiber which transmit "first pain", sharp, prickling and injurious, and C- nerve fibers which responsible for "second pain" dull, aching and visceral. Various chemicals (bradykinin, histamine, serotonin, prostaglandins, potassium, proton) are released into damaged tissue cells of vascular origins (platelets, neutrophils, lymphocytes and macrophages) and also by mast cells. Some of these chemicals induce nociceptive reactions and can modify the activity of nociceptors either by direct activation or by sensitization to different stimuli. Several mediators are involved in this mechanism. They include bradykinin, substances P, cytokines (interleukins, interferon, tumor necrosis factor), nerve growth factor, prostaglandins, leukotriens, galanin, vasoactive intestinal peptide, somatostatin, cholecytokinin, monoamines etc.

Neuropeptides

Neuropeptides include substance P, calitonin gene-related peptide, vasoactive intestinal peptide, nociceptin/orphanin FQ (N/OFQ). Local axon reflexes are responsible for the peripheral release of neuropeptides from sensory neurons leading to neurogenic inflammation [Suzuki et al., 1989]. Primary afferent fibers contained peptides which their profile is altered by sustained stimuli or damage to the nerve [Levine et al., 1993; Hökfelt et al, 1994]. In the spinal horn the peripheral noxious stimulation causes a release not only a substances P but also of other peptides such as neurokinin A (NKA), neurokonin B (NKB), calcitonin gene related peptide (CGRP) and somatostatin but not of galanin [Morton et al., 1988; Morton and Hutchison, 1989].

Substance P

It is synthesized in the spinal ganglion, from where it is transported centrally to the substantia gelatinosa of spinal dorsal horn and peripherally to the nerve endings in many tissues. Substance P occurs in small and medium sized neurons of substantia gelatinosa of the spinal dorsal horns, as well as in peripheral and central endings of primary afferent fibers. It is released by primary afferent nociceptive fibers at the level of spinal cord. It is believed that substance P together with other tachykinins is responsible for nociceptive transmission from the peripheral to the central nervous system [Iversen, 1982]. Intrathecal injection of substance P in mice elicits the behavior suggesting the pain sensation [Hylden and Wilcox, 1981], whereas tachykinin antagonists [Lembeck et al., 1981; Zubrzycka et al., 1997] administered by the same route produce an analgesic effect. Treatment with capsaicin resulted in a decrease in the substance P content in the dorsal horn and concomitant elevation of pain threshold [Nagy and Van Der Kooy, 1983]. The release of substance P is blocked by morphine at trigeminal level [Jessell and Iversen, 1977]. Blocking neurokinin-1 receptor does not alleviate the nociceptive effect of substance P [Mantyh et al., 1995; Mantyh et al., 1997]. Moreover, destruction of the neurons that express neurokinin-1 receptor led to a substantial reduction in allodynia and hyperalgesia induced by inflammation and nerve injury. Substance P appears to have a role in potentiating both excitatory and inhibitory inputs to spinal nociceptive neurons, an effect sensitizing the neurons to any synaptic input [Radhakrishnan and Henry, 1995].

Clinically substance P antagonists failed to relieve the pain in migraine and rheumatoid arthritis [Dray and Rang, 1998]. Substance P plays a role in neurogenic inflammation. It causes a degranulation of mast cells and thus the release of histamine, vasodilatation, and plasma extravasation with the subsequent release of other alogens (serotonin, bradykinin) and the activation of other inflammatory cells (macrophages, lymphocytes). Substance P also is able to induce production of nitric oxide from endothelium. Neurogenic inflammation also involves the release of substance P from sensory nerve endings in response to pain or infection. When the irritant capsaicin was applied to skin, edema occurred as a result of sensory neuropeptide release, including substance P [Iversen, 1998]. Local administration of substance P had no effect on neuronal firing properties [Heppelmann and Pawlak, 1997]. Intense peripheral stimulation may induce release of substance P into the dorsal horn, causing central hyperexcitability and an increased sensitivity to pain [De Felipe et al., 1998]. Substance P and enkephalins exert opposite effects on the nociceptive neurons. Both somatostatin and galanin inhibit the release of substance P [Yangisawa et al., 1986].

Calcitonin Gene Related Peptide (CGRP)

It is derived, with calcitonin, from the CT/CGRP gene located on chromosome 11. It is a 37 amino acid peptide and is the most potent endogenous vasodilator currently known. CGRP was discovered when alternative processing of RNA transcripts from the calcitonin gene was shown to result in the production of distinct mRNAs encoding CGRP [Amara et al., 1982]. It is primarily produced in nervous tissue however its receptors are expressed throughout the body. It is also strongly implicated in the vasodilatory effect of endogenous cannabinoid anandamide in the brain. CGRP enhances the release of substance P from primary afferent neuron [Oku et al., 1987]. CGRP has been shown to be important in the trigeminovascular system that is known to play an important role in the pathogenesis of migraine headache [Edvinsson, 2003; Olesen et al., 2004]. This effect was found to be antagonised by capsazepine [Zygmunt et al., 1999]. In behavioural studies, CGRP has been shown to inhibit the antinociceptive effects produced by opioids [Welch et al., 1989]. Since opioids produce analgesia, in part, by inhibiting the release of sensory transmitters in the spinal cord [Pohl et al., 1989], an adaptative increase in the release of a neuropeptides such as CGRP could physiologically antagonize opioid action and thus lead to the development of tolerance. The combination of a CGRP receptor antagonist with morphine presents an option for the inhibition of clinical tolerance and may provide a new avenue for restoring opioid responsiveness in neuropathic pain states. Hyperresponsivness of sensory neurons following acute synovitis could be blocked by the selective antagonist $CGRP_{8-37}$ [Neugebauer et al., 1996]. Local application of capsaicin onto the sciatic nerve can alleviate mechanical hyperalgesia in a peripheral neuropathic pain models as a result of decrease of TRPV1- and CGRP-positive sensory [Kim et al., 2008]. In the spinal cord, proteasome inhibitors abolished the enhanced capsaicin-evoked calcitonin gene-related peptide (CGRP) release and dynorphin A upregulation, both elicited by nerve injury suggesting the involvement of CGRP in chronic pain [Ossipov et al., 2007].

Tachykinins

Tachykinin peptides are neuropeptides, found from amphibians to mammals. They were so named due to their ability to rapidly induce contraction of gut tissue [Carter and Krause, 1990]. The two human tachykinin genes are called TAC1 and TAC3 for historical reasons, and are equivalent to Tac1 and Tac2 of the mouse, respectively.

The broad term tachykinin refers to a family of neuropeptides that have a common C-terminal amino acid sequence with a varying N-terminal sequence and substance P-like activity. Of the many tachykinins found in nature, only those found in mammals are referred to as neurokinins. In addition to substance P there are other two neurokinins; neurokinin A (NKA) and neurokinin B (NKB) [Vaught, 1988]. Neurokinin A (NKA), formerly known as substance K, is a member of the tachykinin family of neuropeptide neurotransmitters. It is produced from the same preprotachykinin gene as the neuropeptide substance P. The release of NKA by noxious stimuli in the dorsal horn is more widely spread and longer lasting than that of substance P [Duggan et al., 1990].

Neurokinin 1 (NK1) receptors have the greatest affinity for substance P. Substance P is considered to be the primary nociceptive transmitter in afferent sensory fibers, released in response to noxious cutaneous stimuli and participating in conduction across sensory afferent nerves (C-fibers). Selective destruction of neurokinin-1 receptor in the superfacial spinal cord leads to a sustained reduction in allodynia and hyperalgesia induced by inflammation and nerve injury.

Tachykinins include: neurokinin A, neurokinin K, neuropeptide gamma and substance P [Dornan et al., 1993]. There are three known mammalian tachykinin receptors termed NK1, NK2 and NK3. The receptors are not specific to any individual tachykinin, they do have differing affinity for the tachykinins:

NK1: Substance P>Neurokinin A>Neurokinin B

NK2: Neurokinin A > Neurokinin B > Substance P

NK3: Neurokinin B > Neurokinin A > Substance P

Galanin

It is a neuropeptide present in humans and other mammals. It involved in a number of physiological processes including nociception, response to nerve injury and peripheral inflammation [Liu and Hökfelt, 2002] . It is predominantly an inhibitory, hyperpolarizing neuropeptide and as such inhibits neurotransmitter release. It is often co-localized with substance P and calcitonin gene related peptide. Galanin is expressed in dorsal root ganglion at relatively low levels in <5% of small-diameter C fiber type [Hökfelt et al., 1987]. It might play a role in the regulation of inflammation and nociception. The role of galanin in pain signaling is complex. In intact nerves, exogenously applied galanin have both facilitatory and inhibitory effects on nociception [Kuraishi et al., 1991; Post et al., 1988]. Galanin is a strongly inhibitory, hyperpolarizing peptide, which reduces the excitability of its target cells. Galanin, acting at the three galanin receptors, opens ATP-sensitive potassium channels, closes calcium channels (N- and L-types), modifies intracellular calcium levels, reduces the stimulatory effect of muscarinic agonists on phospholipase C and modulates the activity of adenylyl cyclase. Activation of galanin receptor-1 inhibits the release of substance P and alleviates allodynia. Several studies have shown that intrathecal galanin significantly reduces allodynia induced by chronic constriction injury [Liu and Hökfelt, 2000; Yu et al., 1999]. In addition, Eaton et al. [1999] have shown that a spinal cord implant of genetically modified cells that secrete galanin significantly reduces allodynia after chronic constriction injury. It has been found that the concentration of galanin was significantly lower in the ankles and spinal cords of rats with adjuvant arthritis compared to controls [Qinyang et al., 2004].

Vasoactive Intestinal Peptide (VIP)

It is a 28 amino acid neuropeptide that is contained in postganglionic sympathetic as well as capsaicin–sensitive sensory nerve fibers [Ahmed et al., 1995]. VIP6-28 (VIP antagonist) reduced nociceptive and pain levels in rat model of osteoarthritis [McDougall and Watkins, 2006].

Somatosstatin

It is found in cells of dorsal root ganglion and in afferent terminals of the dorsal horn. It released in response to noxious stimuli leading to hyperpolarization and reduced firing rate in dorsal horn cells. Intrathecal administration of somatostatin produces analgesia and motor dysfunction [Mollenholt, 1988].

Endogenous Opioids

Numerous regions of the brain are rich in opioid peptides and the mRNAs for the opioid receptors [Mansour et al., 1996]. The supraspinal actions of opioids have a key role in the analgesic effects of systemic morphine. Moreover, opioids shared in peripheral antinociception in hyperalgesic inflammatory conditions [Stein and Yassouridis, 1997]

Endogenous Cannobinoids

The endocannobinoid anandamide is enzymatically synthesized from free arachidonic acid and ethanolamine [Deutsch and Chin, 1993]. Anandamide is a nonselective ligand that binds to both CB1 and CB2 cannobinoid G-protein-coupled receptors. The activation of these receptors could modulate pain generation and perception [Pertwee, 2001]. Anandamide activates the transient receptor potential vanilloid channel 1 (TRPV1), causing secondary release of CGRP [Zygmunt et al., 1999].

Nociceptin/Orphanin FQ (N/OFQ)

It is an opioid like neuropeptide that has been immunolocalized in the peripheral and central neurons systems where it controls central pain mechanism [Civelli et al., 1998; Darland et al., 1998]. It is able to induce hyperalgesia and allodynia in the joint [McDougall et al., 2006] as a result of secondary release of substance P into the joint. Selective NK1-receptor antagonist RP67580 blocked N/OFQ mediated nociception [McDougall et al., 2001].

Glutamate

It released by primary afferent fibers and had an important role in the spinal mechanisms of pain transmission. Various receptors and subtypes are involved at the spinal level (AMPA, metabotrophic, kainite). The NMDA receptor is important in the synaptic events that lead to central sensitivity and hyperalgesia [Dickenson, 1995; Urban et al., 1994]. The release of substance P into the spinal cord on afferent stimulation removes the magnesium block of the channel of the NMDA-receptor in range of persistent pain state. Activation of NMDA receptors leads to an entry of calcium into the neuron which can then produce other mediators from spinal nerves by increasing the activity of enzymes e.g. nitric oxide synthase, phospholipase A2 [Malmberg and Yaksh, 1992a]

Inhibitory Amino Acids

Glycine and γ-aminobutyric acid (GABA) act at dorsal horn controlling the NMDA receptors and they might play a role in etiology of neuropathic pain. Blockade of spinal GABA or glycine can result in allodynia [Yaksh, 1989]. Up-regulation of spinal GABA receptors occurred when there is peripheral inflammation, to promote inhibition of afferent nociceptive impulses and decrease pain sensation [Dickenson, 1995].

Monoamines

Nociceptive impulses activating the sympathetic nervous system promote norepinephrine releases which in turn accelerates sensitization of the nociceptors creating another vicious cycle [Dray, 1995]. Serotonin is a major inflammatory mediator, especially in the initial phase of inflammatory process [Capasso et al., 1975]. It causes direct activation of sensory neurons via $5HT_3$ receptor activation. As a result of activation of $5HT_2$ and $5HT_3$ receptors, the peripheral nociceptors are activated and producing hyperalgesia and neurogenic inflammation [Richardson et al., 1985; Barnes et al., 1990; Rueff and Dray, 1993]. On the other hand, activation of $5HT_{1B}$ and $5HT_{1D}$ receptors decreases pain and inflammation. In the periphery $5HT_{1B}$ and $5HT_{1D}$ agonists inhibit neurogenic inflammation [Zochodne and Ho, 1994].

Free Radicals

Reactive oxygen species such as hydrogen peroxide, hydroxyl radical are produced by tissue during inflammation. They enhance the effects of bradykinin, prostaglandin E2 and other inflammatory mediators. Nitric oxide has been implicated in the degeneration of intervertebral disc. Elevated nitric oxide production has been found in cerebrospinal fluid in patients with degenerative lumbar disease [Podichetty, 2007]. The level of nitric oxide was significantly higher in the herniated cervical disc specimens obtained from patients undergoing discectomy for persistent radiculopathy compared with the control discs [Kang et al., 1995]. In cervicogenic headache, a unilateral headache that provoked by neck movement or pressure on tender points in the neck, the nitrogen species radicals were significantly elevated in serum during the periods of headache [Inan et al., 2007]. Nitric oxide in a complex way exacerbates the noxious transmission. Intracutaneous injection of nitric oxide provoke pain in human [Holthuusen and Arndt, 1994]. On the other hand topical nitric oxide donor in form of transdermal glyceryl trinitrate preparation improved the clinical outcome of patient with chronic extensor tendinosis at the elbow [Paoloni et al., 2003].

Purines

The receptors for the purines, notably the P2X3 (a ligand-gated ion channel triggered by ATP) which is selectively expressed by small diameter sensory neurons. ATP infusion into trapezius muscle induces strong pain and local tenderness in healthy man. ATP induces sustained facilitation of craniofacial nociception by prolonged excitation of P2X3 receptors in neck muscles [Makowska et al., 2006]. Sole administration of 100 nmol/L ATP facilitates brainstem nociception in mice and it reversed by local application of tetradotoxin in neck muscles [Ellrich and Makowska, 2007].

Bradykinin

It is a powerful alogenic substance released from kininogen in a way that is dependent on protein kinase C and calcium and sensitizes nociceptors by means of activation of postganglionic sympathetic neurons which then produce PGE2. Bradykinin involved in release of prostaglandins, cytokines, free radicals, histamine from degranualted mast cell and stimulation of sympathetic neurons leading to vasodilatation.

Histamine

It is released from mast cells during degranulation, a process promoted by substance P, kinins, interleukin-1, and nerve growth factor. It acts on sensory neurons to produce pain and itching [Simone et al, 1991]. Histamine stimulation of sensory neurons may evoke release neuropeptides and prostaglandins.

Cytokines (Interleukins, Interferon, and Tumor Necrosis Factor)

They are released by phagocytes and cells of the immune system, and have an important role in the inflammatory process. Bradykinin plays a role in the production of cytokines [Dray, 1997]. Some of these cytokines are powerful inflammatory mediators that can activate sensory neuron through different mechanisms, some of which include sympathetic nervous system.

Nerve Growth Factor (NGF)

Central actions, mediated by changes in the expression of neuropeptides, ion channels, and growth factors in the sensory neurons, contribute to later manifestations [Donnerer et al., 1992; Leslie et al., 1995; Michael et al., 1997]. It is upregulated by inflammatory process. It has a key role in the development of sensory and autonomic neuron and process of nociception. It is produced by fibroblast and schwan cells and then increases the excitability of nociceptors which lead to hyperalgesia.

Eicosanoids

Eicosanoids are lipid membrane derived metabolites of arachidonic acid that include prostaglandins, leucotriens, lipoxins, thromboxanes and endocannobinoids. The pain field has generally focused on the activity of cyclooxygenases (COX) of which there are two isoforms COX-1 and COX-2. COX-1 enzyme is constitutively expressed in most cells where its function to maintain normal physiological process in tissues. COX-2 enzyme is present at the site of inflammation (i.e. inducible). Prostaglandins are weak alogens (pain producing) but play major part in the sensitization of receptors to other substances reducing their activation threshold [Birrell et al., 1991; Cohen and Perl, 1990]. Prostaglandin E2 stimulates neurons directly, initiating the transmission of pain impulses along nociceptive pathways. COX -2 enzyme can be produced by different signals mediating cytokines. The antiiinflammatory and antinoceptive effects of COX-2 inhibitors seems to be equivalent to those of non selective COX-2 inhibitors, but the main advantage of COX-2 inhibition will be the absence of gastric side effects in patients with chronic pain of inflammatory origin.

Lipoxins

Lipoxins were first described by Serhan, Hamberg and Samuelsson in 1984. Lipoxins are derived enzymatically from arachidonic acid. Lipoxin, signaling through the lipoxin A4 receptor, inhibits chemotaxis, transmigration, superoxide generation and NF-κB activation (Chiang et al., 2005). Lipoxins are high affinity antagonists to the cysteinyl leukotriene receptor type 1

(CysLT1) to which several leukotrienes (LTC_4, LTD_4 and LTE_4) mediate their smooth muscle contraction and eosinophil chemotactic effects.

Various chemical mediators are involved in turning off inflammation and pain. Lipoxins are one such class mediators that have been formed to act as "braking signals" in inflammation. Lipoxins reduce inflammation when administered directly to the inflamed area or given systematically (intravenously or orally). Acetylsalicylic acid triggers the release of lipoxins as one of its mechanism in reducing inflammation. Lipoxins have central and peripheral effects. Svensson et al [2007] showed that intravenous or intraspinal lipoxins injections can alter pain processing and reduce the pain sensitivity in rats. Local anti-inflammatory effect is observed with intravenous lipoxins injection.

Lipoxin A_4 and aspirin-triggered lipoxin A_4 are anti- inflammatory, proresolving possess, and modulate leukotrienes, cytokines, and chemokines [Serhan, 2005]. LXA_4 and its receptor are present in human osteoarthritis and synovitis of rheumatoid arthritis [Marcouiller et al., 2005; Hashimoto et al., 2007]. Human synovial fibroblasts express LXA, and, at nano- molar concentrations, LXA_4 reduces the levels of inflammatory cytokines and matrix metalloproteinases in synovial fibroblasts stimulated with interleukin 1β, as well as stimulating tissue inhibitors of metalloproteinase- 1[Sodin-Semrl, 2000;2004].

Resolvins and Protectins

These compounds are made by the human body from the omega-3 fatty acids eicosapentaenoic acid and docosahexaenoic acid. They are produced by the COX-2 pathway especially in the presence of aspirin. These mediators have anti-inflammatory and pro-resolution properties, thereby protecting organs from collateral damage, stimulating the clearance of inflammatory debris and promoting mucosal antimicrobial defense [Serhan et al., 2008]. Experimental evidence indicates that resolvins reduce cellular inflammation by inhibiting the production and transportation of inflammatory cells and chemicals to the sites of inflammation. Resolvin E1, at very low amounts reduces polymorph nuclear cells migration, dermal inflammation and interleukin-12 production [Serhan et al., 2002; Arita et al., 2005]. Resolvins and protectins transforming growth factor-β and growth factors produced by macrophages, also have a crucial role in the resolution of inflammation, including the initiation of tissue repair [Serhan and Savill, 2005; Serhan, 2007].

Ions Channel Ligands

Multiple different types of ion channels exist on the terminals of nociceptors. They are activated either directly or via coupling process. These channels:

a   *Acid sensing ion channel.* Acid sensing ion channel closely match the proton-gated cation channel described in sensory neurons. It is expressed in dorsal root ganglia and is also distributed widely throughout the brain. It is rapidly activated by condition of acidity below pH 6.5 [Waldmann et al., 1997].

b   *Sodium channel.* Up-regulation of sodium channels expression is observed in chronic inflammation [Black et al., 2004]. Inflammatory mediators (PGs, adenosine, 5HT) augment the sodium channel kinetics and tetrodotoxin-resistant current [England et al., 1996]. These mediators facilitate transmission of action potentials by modification of the voltage threshold of several ion channels including the tetrodotoxin–resistant sodium channels. Therefore sodium channel blockers like mexilitine and crobenetine inhibit mechanical hyperalgesia [Laird et al., 2001].

c   *TRP channel.* Of particular interest in pain research are TRPM (melanostatin) and the TRMV (vanilloid) channels subfamilies. The eight member of the TRPM channel (TRPM8) is activated by cooling temperature (22-26°C). Pharmacological activation of TRPM8 channel could elicit an antinociceptive effect. The ion channel responsible for noxious thermo-sensation is TRPV1 [Caterina et al., 1997]. TRPV1-channel is activated by temperature above 43°C, proton, lipids, phorbols and cannobinoids. Capsaicin sensitizes afferent neurons by secondary release of inflammation peptides.

Chapter III

Central, Topical and Peripherally Acting Analgesics

Several drug categories are included in the management of neck pain. Their effects are either centrally or peripherally or sometimes at both levels. The majority of these drugs are prescribed to alleviate pain and muscle spasm or to stabilize the nerve function. In certain occasion, drugs combination is prescribed for the purpose of synergism and in other situation intrathecal injection is necessary to combat the neck pain. The following drug categories are currently used in the management of neck pain:

A. Nonsteroidal Anti-Inflammatory Drugs (NSAIDs)

The prostaglandins are implicated in various physiological and pathophysiological events. The prostanoid family includes PGD2, PGE2, PGF2α, Thromboxane A2 and prostaglandins. The biosynthesis of prostaglandins and some other prostanoids is catalyzed in a rate limiting step by PG-H synthase (COX), PG-endoperoxidase synthase which converts arachidonic acid to prostaglandin/prostanoid precursor PGH2. More than three cyclogenases isoenzymes are characterized. These are:

COX-1 (human 576aa, 69-72kDa; chromosome 9), COX-2 (human, 604aa, 74 kDa ; chromosome 1), COX-3 (canine 633aa, 65kDa in human aorta), COX-1 derived-proteins or partial COX-1 (PCOX1a; canine 414aa, 53kDa in human aorta and PCOX1b).

COX-1, a constitutively expressed isoform, produces physiologically relevant prostanoids such as in stomach and platelets. COX-2 is inducible and rapidly up-regulated at inflammation sites and forms proinflammatory prostanoids (Box 2). Prostanoids sensitize peripheral nociceptor terminals and produce localized pain hypersensitivity

In 1971, professor John Vane from Cornell University was awarded the Nobel Prize for his work in elucidating the mechanism of action of aspirin on prostaglandins [cited from Marienfeld et al., 1997]. Nonsteroidal anitiinflammatory drugs reduce the formation of prostaglandins by inhibiting the activity of COX-1, COX-2 and COX-3.

Box 2. Expression of COX isoform enzymes

Arachidonic acid		
COX-1	COX-2	COX-3
Prostaglandins production		
Gastric protection Platelet activation	Inducible inflammation	Pain and fever

Possible effects (mechanisms) for the analgesic activity of NSAIDs include:

1. Peripheral actions via:

- Altering stimulation of sensory nerve endings. NSAIDs reduce prostaglandins production leading to block the nociception response to endogenous mediators of inflammation, with the effect being greater in tissues that have been subjected to injury and trauma [Kitahata, 1993]. Also they inhibit prostaglandin-mediated sensitization of nociceptors to chemical and mechanical irritants [Dahl and Kehlet, 1991].
- Interfering with membrane signal transduction. They stabilize the cell membrane, an effect may account for the decrease in prostaglandins release.
- Interfering with bradykinin activity.

2. Central actions via:

- Interfering with prostaglandins synthesis.
- Altering transmission of impulses by nerves that release substance P or CGRP.
- Causing the release of endogenous opioid (enkephalin) or GABA, leading to impulse transmission block.
- Intrathecal adminstration of NSAIDs have been shown to reduce hyperalgesia [Malmberg and Yaksh, 1992b]. NSAIDs affect the synthesis of substances thought to play role in the processing of nociceptive impulses in the dorsal horn like serotonin, kynuremic acid and polyamines [McCormack, 1994].

3. Other possible mechanisms of action of NSAIDs in inhibiting inflammation:

1. Alter neutrophil function.
2. Interfere with mitochondrial function, alters oxidative phosphorylation, decrease ATP.
3. Stabilize lysosomal membranes.
4. Interfere with kinin formation and/or activity.
5. Inhibit the activity of selecins.
6. Inhibit NF-kB formation (NF-kB is important in production and stimulation of cytokines)

Classification of COX Inhibitors (Tables 1 and 2)

1. Selective COX-1: COX-1 inhibitors with not measurable effects of COX-2 activity e.g. low doses of acetylsalicylic acid (potent inhibitor at concentration 0.1 mM). Sodium salicylate is very weak inhibitor of COX-1.
2. Nonselective COX: Minimal differences between dose-response curves inhibition of either COX-1 or COX-2.
3. Preferential COX-2: It appears to produce its pharmacological effects on COX-2 at doses that have minimal effects on COX-1. However, high doses inhibit COX-1.

4. Selective COX-2: It only inhibits COX-2 at maximum therapeutic dose. Increasing dose should not result in significant inhibition of COX-1.

Table 1. IC_{50} values for the inhibition of COX-1 and COX-2 in human whole blood assay

Drug	IC_{50} (COX-1) µM	IC_{50} (COX-2) µM	COX-1/COX-2 ratio
Indomethacin	0.19	0.44	0.4
Ibuprofen	4.8	24.3	0.2
6-MNA metabolite	28.9	154	0.2
Piroxicam	0.76	9.0	0.2
Etodolac	9.0	3.7	2.4
Meloxicam	1.4	7.0	2.0
Diclofenac	0.15	0.05	3.0
Celecoxib	6.7	0.87	7.7
Valdecoxib	26.1	0.87	30
Etoricoxib	116	1.1	106

Table 2. IC_{50} values for the inhibition of COX-1 and COX-2 in intact cells

Drug	IC_{50} (COX-1) µM	IC_{50} (COX-2) µM	COX-1/COX-2 ratio
Acetylsalicylic acid	1.67	278	166
Sulindac	1.12	112	100
Indomethacin	0.03	1.68	60
Sodium salicylate	254	725	2.8
Acetaminophen	17.9	133	2.4
Valdecoxib	26.1	0.87	0.03

The following general notes should be taken in consideration when NSAIDs are prescribed to patients with neck pain:

1. They reduce pain at low doses and decrease inflammation at high doses.
2. Once-a-day dosing is preferable to improve compliance.
3. Salicylic acid in pharmaceutical preparation of aspirin is rarely indicated because an irreversible inhibition of cyclooxygeneases.
4. All NSAIDs have a dose-related ceiling point for analgesia.
5. The efficacy of COX-2 inhibitors is the same with the noselective inhibitors.

NSAIDs in lower dosages and a less regular schedule is more likely to utilize the analgesic properties. In single dose, most of NSAIDs are effective analgesics than a single dose of acetaminophen or acetylsalicylic acid. The analgesic actions of NSAIDs can be dissociated from the anti-inflammatory effect, and this may reflect additional spinal and supraspinal actions of NSAIDs to inhibit various aspect of central pain processing [Yaksh et al., 1998]. Both COX- isoforms (COX-1 and COX-2) contribute to spinal and supraspinal prostanoid production following tissue injury or inflammation [Yaksh et al., 1998]. Moreover, NSAIDs had effect upon the healing of the injured soft tissue, namely muscle and tendon. In vitro model of isolated human fibroblast subjected to repeated motion injury, indomethacin accelerates the protein synthesis during the later remodeling phase of healing [Almekinders et al., 1995].

Celecoxib, COX-2 inhibitor, showed better scores than sustained release acetaminophen for pain, stiffness and functional limitation in patients with osteoarthritis in multiple sites [Yelland et al., 2006]. COX-2 inhibitors have been associated with cardiovascular toxicity. Rofecoxib was withdrawn from the worldwide market because of this effect, demonstrated in the APPROVE trial. This trial was conducted at 108 centers worldwide with recruitment in 2000 and 2001, and examined the protective effect of rofecoxib on adenomatous polyps but was terminated early because of cardiovascular toxicity [Baron et al., 2008]. The use of 25 mg/day rofecoxib is associated with increased risk for cardiovascular event which persists to one year after treatment is stopped.

Topical NSAIDs

When NSAIDs are administered topically, relatively high concentrations occur in the dermis, where levels in the muscle are at least equivalent to those following systemic administration [Heyneman et al., 2000]. Topically applied NSAIDs do reach the synovial fluid, but it is not clear whether this effect reflect local penetration or results from systemic circulation [Vaile and Davis, 1998]. In human topical application of NSAIDs produces analgesia in models of cutaneous pain [McCormack et al., 2000] and muscle pain [Steen et al., 2000]. The effect of topical NSAIDs in osteoarthritis and rheumatoid arthritis varied between 18-92% [Heyneman et al., 2000].

Topical application of NSAIDs may be useful for acute inflammation and localized pain. In experimental animal model patch sheets of loxoprofen sodium, felbinac, indomethacin or ketoprofen have analgesic effects, inhibit expression of c-Fos in the dorsal horn (loxoprofen sodium and indomethacin), and reduce PGE2 levels (loxoprofen sodium in inflamed tissues [Sekiguchi et al., 2008]. Adverse reactions of topical NSAIDs are cutaneous which occur in 10-15% of patient in form of skin rash and pruritis at the site of application [Moore et al., 1998] and less likely systemic adverse reactions.

B. Acetaminophen; The Para-Amino Phenol Derivative

It is the active metabolite of phenacetin a so called coal tar analgesic. In vivo, phenacetin is converted to acetaminophen. In 1852 Gerhardt discovered acetaminophen that reducing fever and pain. It was first used in clinical medicine in 1893 but wide spread use began after its FDA approval in 1950. It is effective as an analgesic and antipyretic. It has a weak anti-inflammatory action; possibly due to its weak inhibition of cyclooxygenase (as measured in the presence of high concentrations of peroxides found in inflammatory lesions) and hence its weak inhibition of prostaglandin synthesis. Acetaminophen has a unique activity profile based in part on its action at its molecular targets, the cyclooxygenase enzyme that produces prostaglandins responsible for pain, fever and inflammation. COX-3 (a COX enzyme isoform encoded by COX-1 gene) is sensitive to selective inhibition by acetaminophen that reduces pain and fever but has weak anti-inflammatory (Chandrasekharan et al., 2002; Warner and Mitchel, 2002). Therefore, its efficacy as an analgesic may be less than other nonsteroidal anti-inflammatory drugs like aspirin. COX-3 is also the target for diclofenac, aspirin and ibuprofen.

In therapeutic doses, acetaminophen inhibits the activity of COX-3 enzyme while in toxic doses it activates nuclear receptor (CAR) leading to expression of three cytochrome P450 enzymes that transform acetaminophen into a reactive toxic metabolites, NAPOI which responsible for hepatotoxicity. Acetaminophen is primarily centrally acting, has no effect on platelet aggregation, and is reversible inhibitor of cyclooxygenase enzyme. In experimental animal model, pretreatment of rats with oral acetaminophen significantly attenuated intrathecal substance P-induced hyperalgesia and suppressed the release of spinal PGE2 [Crawley et al., 2008]. Also intrathecal acetaminophen produces dose dependent antinoceptive effect indicating the central hyperalgesic action of acetaminophen. The antipyretic activity is exerted by blocking the effect of endogenous pyrogens on the hypothalamic heat-regulation center possibly by inhibiting prostaglandins synthesis. Analgesic effect of acetaminophen may be produced by direct action on the pain threshold. This effect is believed to be due to inhibition of prostaglandins and/or inhibition of the synthesis or actions of chemical mediators or other substances that sensitize the pain receptors to mechanical or chemical stimulation.

It is the preferred analgesic for patients with osteoarthritis and other conditions associated with minor pain. One survey estimated that nearly 3% of all Americans over 20 years old are frequent monthly users of acetaminophen [Paulose-Ram et al., 2005].

Acetaminophen is being more effective than placebo in relieving pain of large joint osteoarthritis but NSAIDs and coxibs show superior efficacy to acetaminophen and are also effective for stiffness [Neame et al., 2004; Zhang et al., 2004; Pincus et al., 2004].

The hazard ratio for hospitalization for a gastrointestinal event was 1.2 for patients taking more than 3g /day acetaminophen; 1.63 for those taking NSAIDs and 2.55 for those taking combination of NSAIDs and more than 3g/day of acetaminophen [Rahme et al., 2008]. Acetaminophen is able to exert analgesic effect in nociceptive tests that are sensitive to central analgesics and in which there is no inflammation [Bustamante et al., 1996]. In the rat formalin test, significant reduction in the antinoceceptive action of acetaminophen is observed when the serotonergic bulbospinal pathways are damages or there is depletion in serotonin level [Pini et al., 1996]. Intrathecal administration of 5HT receptor antagonists inhibit the antinociceptive action of acetaminophen suggesting that the inhibition occurred as the spinal level by means of a serotonergic mechanism [Courade et al ., 2001]. Moreover, intrathecal injection of selective $5HT_{A1}$ receptor antagonist (WAY-100635) reversed the action of acetaminophen in the rat formalin test suggesting that its antinociceptive activity depends on the stimulation of the spinal $5HT_{A1}$ receptor [Bonnefont et al., 2003; 2005]. Bonnefont et al [2007] showed that specific 5-HT_{A1} receptor-dependent cellular events in acetaminophen produced antinociception, and the inhibition of COX activities is not the exclusive mechanism involved.

C. Opioids

Presynaptic opioid receptors decrease the release of excitatory neurotransmitters from nociceptive neurons, specifically the neurons that send small C-fibers and Aδ fibers into the periphery and respond to a variety of noxious stimuli. Postsynaptic opioid receptors have similar effects on the second-order neuron. Opioids exert their analgesic effects by binding to and activating receptors that comprise part of an endogenous opioid system. There are three distinct families of endogenous opioid peptides: the endorphins (interact with μ and δ receptors), the enkephalins (interact with δ receptors), and the dynorphins (interact with κ receptors). Also two additional short peptides that display a high affinity and selectivity for μ opioid receptors have been identified. These peptides; endomorphin-1 and endomorphin-2, produce potent and prolonged analgesia in animals. Most recently, a receptor that is structurally similar to the opioid receptor was discovered. This receptor has been classified as opioid-receptor-like 1 (ORL1). The natural ligand has been termed orphanin FQ (OFQ), or nociceptin. It appears to be involved in the central modulation of pain. Opioid receptors that are capable of mediating analgesia in humans have been discovered on peripheral sensory nerve terminals and are very similar to those of receptors in the brain. The prevailing peptides found in the periphery are the endorphins and enkephalins. This peripheral opioid system interacts with immune functions. In brief the supraspinal and peripheral analgesia produced by opioid are related to:

1. *mu*-and/or δ receptor agonists reduce release primary afferent neurotransmitters (substance P, glutamate) from C-fibers and inhibited the release of CGRP [Dickenson,1986; Kangrga and Randić, 1991].
2. *mu*-receptor agonists prevent the nociceptor sensitization by PGE2 by μ-receptor agonist [Levine and Taiwo, 1989]. Also delta and kappa receptor agonists block bradykinin-induced release of nocoiceptor sensitizing agents from the nerve ending [Taiwo and Levine, 1991]. Intraarticular injection of morphine before the procedure of arthroscopy appears to be more effective than after arthroscopy. This supports the importance of preemptive inhibition of peripheral inflammatory and hyperalgesia pathway [Denti, 1997]. Topical application of opioid to somatic site may also produces analgesia in number of experimental models [Nozaki-Taguchi and Yaksh, 1999].

3. Opioid will delay the onset of wind-up phenomenon.
4. Antiinflammatory property, opioids reduced the synovial leucocytes count, may have contributed to the pain relief [Martinez et al., 1996].

Opioids are very effective in reducing the severity of spine pain and in producing pain relief. Dosage escalations are typically related to an identifiable worsening of the painful condition, a surgical complication or an unrelated pain process [Mahowald et al., 2005].

Oxycodone (controlled release) therapy significantly improved the quality of life and quality of sleep in patients with refractory and frequent acute episodes of chronic neck pain who failed to respond to non-opioid conservative treatment [Ma et al., 2007]. Patients with chronic neck pain due to facet cervical joint pain were responded to fentanyl better than midazolam sedation [Manchikanti et al., 2004a]. Chao et al [2005] observed that oral morphine (sustained release) reduced the main pain score in patients with lower back pain with radiculoneuropathy, neck pain, headache, degenerative disc disease, failed back syndrome, and radiculoneuropathies and its use did not result in escalation of dose strength or frequency, and was safe and efficacious regardless of patient age. Small-dose ketamine improved the analgesic effects of fentanyl patient controlled analgesia after cervical surgery and to a less extent after lumbar surgery [Yamauchi et al., 2008]. The quality of emergence from anesthesia in patients with cervical spine surgery is improved with fentanyl-based anesthesia [Inoue et al., 2005].

Opioid therapy should be considered in severe cervical spondylosis as the preferred treatment since of addiction during therapy is less than 1%.

Long term opioid treatment for nonmalignant pain is not appropriate for the large majority of patients, and that most patients do worse, not better [Schofferman, 1993].

Transdermal Fentanyl

Use of transdermal fentanyl in chronic non malignant pain is controversial. Patients with low back pain can be successfully given transdermal fentanyl with similar or improved control pain [Jeal and Benfield, 1997]. Data from open, randomized, parallel group multicenter study included 680 patients with chronic low back pain showed that transdermal fentanyl and sustained release morphine provided similar levels of pain relief besides that transdermal fentanyl is associated with significantly less constipation than sustained release morphine [Allan et al., 2005]. Patients with neuropathic pain temporarily responded to intravenous fentanyl and good prolonged pain control with tolerable side effects [Dellemijn and Vanneste, 1997]. In a 16-week open-label study evaluated pre- and postdrug therapy effects, Agarwal et al [2007] found that significant reduction in pain intensity and increase in daytime activity in chronic neuropathic pain patients treated with transdermal fentanyl.

Opioid and Dependence

Neck pain was estimated in relation to analgesic consumption at baseline. Individuals who reported use of analgesics daily or weekly at baseline showed significant increased risk for having chronic pain and analgesic overuse at follow-up but it was less evident than individuals with chronic migraine [Zwart et al., 2003]. Persons with chronic spinal pain were at elevated risk to have chronic pain at other anatomic sites, to have a range of medical comorbidities, and to have mood and substance use disorders [Gureje et al., 2007].

Chronic pain and prolonged use of opioids raise the prevalence of opioids dependence in spine surgery patients to 20% [Walid et al., 2007]. In that study, thirty patients were opioid dependent among 150 spine surgery patients [48 lumbar diskectomy, 60 cervical decompression and fusion and 42 lumbar decompression and fusion]. And the prevalence was highest among lumbar decompression and fusion patients and among females, and was positively correlated with pain intensity. Opioid tolerance to the peripheral analgesia may developed [Aley et al., 1995], and it reversed or even prevented by NMDA receptor antagonists [Kolensnikov and Pasternak, 1999]. Studies of opioids for nonmalignant pain have shown minimal risk of addiction or abuse behaviors in patients with neuropathic pain [Watson and Babul, 1998].

On the other hand narcotic abuse is considered as a cause of neck pain. There is a high risk of cervical osteomyelitis in intravenous drug abusers due to the use of jugular veins for administration of drugs. Rapid vertebral body destruction at any cervical levels secondary to cervical osteomyelitis in an intravenous drug abuser was reported [Arun et al., 2007; Singh et al., 2006]. Advanced vertebral body destruction, disk space infection, prevertebral abscess, and anterior cervical inflammatory reaction appear to be typical findings on radiographs in heroin abusers with cervical osteomyelitis [Endress et al., 1990]. Schreiber and Formal [2007] reported spinal cord infarction in the anterior spinal artery distribution in woman recreationally inhaled cocaine presented with neck pain and muscle weakness.

D. Capsaicinoids and Vanilloids Agonists

Capsaicin
Dihydrocapsaicin
Nordihydrocapsaicin
Homodihydrocapsaicin
Homocapsaicin
Nonivamide

Capsaicin

Capsaicin is the active component of chili peppers which are plants belonging to the genus Capsicum. It produces burning sensation in any tissue with which comes in contact. Pure capsaicin is a hydrophobic, colorless, odorless, crystalline- waxy compound. It was first isolated in 1816 in crystalline form by P.A. Bucholz and again 30 years later by L.T. Thresh who give it the name capsaicin. It was first synthesized in 1930 by E. Spath and F.S. Darling. In 1961, similar substances were isolated from chili peppers by the Japanese chemists S. Kosuge and Y. Inagaki who named them capsaicinoids [Kosuge et al., 1961; Kosuge and Inagaki 1962].

Capsaicin is currently used in topical ointments to relieve the pain of peripheral neuropathy (postherpetic neuralgia). It may be used as creams for the temporarily relief of minor aches and pains of muscles and joints associated with arthritis, simple backache, strains and sprains. Recently it is used to prevent post-operative pain.

Capsaicin binds to Transient Receptor Potential Vanilloid Type 1 (TRPV1) receptor. Vanilloid receptor type 1 is a member of the transient receptor potential family of ion channels, is a modestly calcium-selective ion channel located in C-fiber and Aδ sensory neurons as well as in a growing number of other sites such as the central nervous system or the bladder [Szallasi, 2001] and when activated produces desensitization or degeneration of the sensory afferent. Mice deficient of TRPV1 show impaired pain response to heat [Caterina et al., 2000]. Capsaicin is a heat activated calcium channel with a threshold to open between 37°C and 45°C, causes the channel to lower its opening threshold, thereby opening it at temperatures less than the body's temperature that is why capsaicin is linked to the sensation of heat. Weisman et al [1994] reported that topical capsaicin (0.075%) for six weeks produced a reduction in inflammatory mediators including substances P in synovial fluid of patients with rheumatoid arthritis. Botulinium toxin A suppressed the trigeminal/cervical nociceptive system (hyperalgesia and vasomotor activity) activated by intradermal injection of capsaicin to the forehead of healthy subjected [Gazerani et al., 2006]. Prolonged activation of these neurons by capsaicin depletes presynaptic substance P. There is evidence that capsaicin interacted with tetradotoxin in favor of synergism to suppress the thermal nociception [Kohane et al., 1999]. Neurons that do not contain TRPV1 are unaffected. The rationale for the topical application of capsaicin and other vanilloids in the treatment of pain is that such compounds selectively excite and subsequently desensitize nociceptive neurons. This desensitization is triggered by the activation of vanilloids receptor (TRPV1) which leads to an elevation in intracellular calcium level. The application of vanilloid agonists to the peripheral nerves provide conduction blockade. This is not associated with suppression of motor or sensory functions not related to pain as with a local anaesthetic. Fitzgerald and Woolf [1982] reported that capsaicin (1.5%) applied locally to a peripheral nerve provided inhibition of responses to noxious heat stimuli for up to 16 days, but noxious mechanical stimuli were unaffected by this treatment. Topical capsaicin preparations (0.025-0.075%) are available for human use and produces benefit in postherpetic neuralgia, diabetic neuropathy, postmastectomy pain syndrome, oral neuropathic pain, trigeminal neuralgia, tempromandibular joint disorder, cluster headache and osteoarthritis. Capsaicin is not satisfactory for chronic pain, and is often adjuvant to other approaches [Watson, 1994].

Homocapsaicin

It is a capsaicinoid and analog and congener of capsaicin in chili peppers (*Capsicum*). It accounts for about 1% of the total capsaicinoids mixture and has about half the pungency of capsaicin. It is a lipophilic colorless odorless crystalline to waxy compound.

Resiniferatoxin

Resiniferatoxin (RTX), isolated from *Euphorbia resinifera*, is a natural product in which the alkyl C-region of capsaicin is replaced with a tricyclic diterpene structurally related to those found in the phorbol esters. It is much more potent than capsaicin [Szallasi et al., 1999]. In experimental animal it produced a long standing thermal and mechanical hypoalgesia with a very wide separation between effective concentrations (0.00003-0.001%), providing an effect lasting from several hours to several weeks. Xu et al., [1997] reported that the systemic administration of RTX (0.5 mg/kg subcutaneously) caused a marked thermal hypoalgesia that started to recover after two weeks and also caused mechanical hypoalgesia, which recovered a week after the injection. Systemic injection of RTX destroys TRPV1-expressing sensory neurons and induces a long-lasting impairment of thermal nociception in adult rats [Pan et al., 2003]. Percutaneous administration of RTX to peripheral nerves can provide long-lasting suppression, not only thermal but also mechanical nociception [Kissin et al., 2002]. Resiniferatoxin-induced conduction blockade has an inherent drawback of TRPV1 agonist, the initial excitation (pain) [Kissin, 2008].

E. Neurotoxins

Cervical dystonia, also called spasmodic torticollis, is the third most common movement disorder, after Parkinson's disease and tremor, affecting approximately 125,000 people in the United States. The symptoms of cervical dystonia usually develop gradually over a period of time, with the severity of symptoms leveling off after five years. This excessive muscle activity is often painful. In one study of 170 patients, more than 90 percent of cervical dystonia patients experienced chronic pain [Zesiewicz et al., 2004]. Neurotoxins are currently used to treat this condition.

Botulinum Toxin

Botulinum toxin is a neurotoxin produced by *Clostridium botulinum*, spore-forming anaerobic bacillus. It cleaves synaptic vesicle association membrane protein (synaptobrevin) which is a component of the protein complex responsible for docking and fusion of the synaptic vesicle to the presynaptic membrane. It blocks acetylcholine release and then paralyzes the muscle for 3-4 months.

In December 1989, botulinium toxin A was approved by the US Food and Drug Administration (FDA) for the treatment of strabismus, blepharospasm, and hemifacial spasm in patients over 12 years old. Botulinium toxin A (Botox) is approved by FDA for treating severe spasm of neck muscle and severe primary axillary hyperhidrosis. Botulinium Toxin Type B (Myobloc) received FDA approval for treatment of cervical dystonia on December, 2000. The specific biological activity for (Botox) is 60 MU-Ev/ng neurotoxin, for Dysport 10 MU-Ev/ng neurotoxin, and for Myobloc/Neurobloc 5 MU-EV/ng neurotoxin. Botulinium toxin A or B indicated for cervical dystonia when all of the following criteria are met:

- There are clonic and/or tonic involuntary contractions of multiple neck muscles.
- There is sustained head torsion and/or tilt with with limited range of motion in the neck.
- Duration of the condition is greater than six months.
- Secondary causes of dystonia are excluded e.g. chronic neuroleptic syndrome, contractures or other neuro-muscular disorders.

Botulinium toxin A is effective therapy for neck muscle spasm (cervical dystonia) and myofacial neck pain (Sycha et al., 2004). Acute-onset posttraumatic cervical dystonia is poorly responded to botulinium toxin A injections [Tarsy, 1998].

Botulinium injections reduced motor end plate activity and the interference pattern of electromyography significantly but had no effect on either pain (spontaneous or referred) or pain thresholds compared with isotonic saline [Qerama et al., 2006]. The findings of Qerama et al., study are in agreement with Ojala et al., study [2006] who found in a double blind, randomized, controlled cross-over study that there was no difference between the effect of small doses of botulinium toxin A and those of the physiological saline in the treatment of myofacial pain syndrome as well as Ferrante et al [2005] who, in randomized, double blind, placebo controlled study, reported that injection of botulinium toxin A directly into trigger points did not improve cervico-thoracic myofascial pain.

Freund and Schwartz (2000) reported a significant improvement in objective of total range of neck motion and subjective pain in patients with whiplash associated disorder. The effect of botulinum toxin A persists for several weeks and neck weakness is the adverse reaction of such therapy (Bihari, 2005). Subsequent treatment is associated with no therapeutic response in 5-10% i.e. resistance due to formation of blocking antibodies (Klein, 2002). Single intramuscular injection of botulinium toxin sero B relieved the pain of cervical dystonia in patients who poorly responded to botulinium toxin A (Costa et al.,2004). Injection of botulinum toxin A into neck extensor musculature may cause rapidly progressive cervical kyphosis [Hogan et al., 2006]

Antibodies can develop after repeated use of high doses of botulinium toxin A in some individuals, making further treatment ineffective indefinitely. Because of unique mechanism of action and antigenicity of botulinium toxin A, it may be effective in patients with cervical dystonia who developed antibodies or who have not responded to botulinium toxin B. An estimated 5-15% of patients with injected serially with 79-11 Botox developed secondary non-responsiveness from the production of neutralizing antibodies. Risk factors associated with the development of neutralizing antibodies include injection of more than 200 units per session and repeated a booster injection given within one month of treatment. The new BCB 2024 Botox may have a lower potential for neutralizing antibody production because of its decreased protein load. Antibodies are produced in association with certain treatment parameters, patients'characteristics and immunological properties of the botulinium toxin preparation used [Dressler and Hallett, 2006]. For myobloc/Neurobloc, this translates into an antibody-induced therapy failure rate of 44% in patients treated for cervical dystonia whereas for BTX-A preparation this figure is approximately 5%.

F. Alpha-2 Adrenoceptor Agonists

α_2-adrenoceptor agonists are nonspecific analgesics. Although the overall response rate appears to be only fair, some patients clearly benefit. Potentially, any type of pain may be treated with these drugs. Injection of α_2-adrenoceptor agonists along axon has been suggested to improve the nerve block characteristics of local anesthetic solution through either a local vasoconstriction [Gaumann et al., 1992], a facilitation of C-fiber blockade from the local anesthetic solution [Gaumann et al., 1994] or spinal action cause by slow retrograde axonal transport or single diffusion along the nerve [Brimijoin and Helland, 1976].

Tizanidine

It is related to centrally acting skeletal muscle relaxant. It is α_2-agonist adrenergic receptor presumably reduces spasticity by increasing presynaptic inhibition of motor neurons. The effects of tizanidine are greatest on polysynaptic pathways.

It can be effective for tension headache, back pain, neuropathic pain and myofascial pain. Although clonidine has been used for refractory neuropathic pain, tizanidine tended to be better tolerated than clonidine and unlike clonidine, rarely decreased blood pressure. The sedative property of tizanidine may benefit patients with insomnia caused by severe muscle spasm [See and Ginsburg, 2008]. Tizanidine is used to relieve the spasms and increased muscle tone caused by multiple sclerosis, stroke, or brain spinal injury. It is indicated for treating muscle spasm in patients with cervical strain. Tizanidine as baclofen may have less potential for addiction.

Clonidine

The addition of clonidine to local anesthetic solution improved peripheral nerve blockade by reducing the onset time, extending postoperative analgesia and improving the efficacy of nerve block during surgery [Bernard and Macarie, 1997; Salonen et al., 1992]

In the double blind study by De Kock [1999], an infusion of clonidine 6 mg/kg/hr reduced intra-opertaive intravenous propofol and post-opertaive analgesic requirements, with only asymptomatic bradycardia. Further double-blind, placebo controlled trial by Murga et al [1994], intra-operative requirements of fentanyl is reduced by 50% and provided post-operative analgesia for hours without significant reduced blood pressure.

G. NMDA- Receptor Antagonists

There are several drugs that block NMDA receptor. All these drugs are used now to treat neuropathic pain. These drugs include: dextromethorphan, amantadine, memantine and ketamine.

Dextromethorphan

Dextromethorphan is a low-affinity, noncompetitive *N*-methyl-D-aspartate (NMDA) receptor antagonist used to treat a variety of painful conditions. It inhibits both wind-up and NMDA receptor-mediated nociceptive responses of secondary-order neurons within the spinal cord dorsal horn [Dickenson et al., 1991; Tal and Bennett, 1993].

In one placebo-controlled, double-blind, randomized crossover study, single dose (270 mg) of dextromethophan hydrobromide produced a statistically significant analgesic effect, compared with placebo, in patients with post-traumatic neuropathic pain [Carlsson et al., 2004]. In randomized, double-blind, crossover trial, oral dextromethorphan for 6 weeks had no significant analgesic effect in pain due to possible trigeminal neuropathy and anesthesia dolorosa [Gilron et al .,2000].

Amantadine

Amantadine is an NMDA receptor antagonist which may help prevent the central nervous system changes associated with chronic pain that make chronic pain difficult to treat. Amantadine was originally developed as an anti-viral medication and has been also used to treat Parkinson's disease. In experimental randomized, blinded, and placebo controlled study, Lascelles et al [2008] demonstrated that the addition of amantadine to meloxicam improved the physical activity of dogs with refractory osteoarthritic pain. It is an attractive "third man in" for patients inadequately managed on NSAIDs and tramadol or it can be teamed with an opioid alone (tramadol or oral morphine) in NSAID, intolerant patients.

Memantine

Although NMDA receptors play a substantial role in central nervous system changes underlying neuropathic pain, Wiech et al [2004] found that memantine a NMDA receptor antagonist had no effect on the intensity of chronic phantom limb pain.

Ketamine

Treatment options for patients with chronic persistent pain, who received narcotic analgesia, include dose escalation, opioid rotation, drug holidays, and the addition of adjuvants. Some experts advocate the use of NMDA-receptor antagonists to combat tolerance. The effect of ketamine on neuropathic pain seems to be more potent than that of dextromethorphan [Mao, 2002]. Intravenous ketamine test may be a valuable tool in predicting subsequent response to dextromethorphan treatment in opioid-exposed patients [Cohen et al 2004]. No significant differences in the response to either ketamine or dextromethorphan treatment based on pain classification (i.e., nociceptive, neuropathic, or mixed) or placebo response [Cohen et al., 2008].

H. Muscle Relaxants

Muscle relaxants are thought to be useful in pain disorders based on the theory that pain induces spasm and spasm causes pain. Central muscle relaxants act as sedatives which most likely cause their muscle relaxant effects. They are commonly used to treat muscle spasms in the neck pain. Spasmolytics like carisoprodol, cyclobenzaprine, metaxalone and methocarbamol, are commonly prescribed for low back pain or neck pain, fibromyalgia, tension headache and myofascial pain syndrome. They are not more effective than paracetamol or non-steroidal anti-inflammatory drugs, and in fibromyalgia they are not more effective than antidepressants [Chou et al., 2007; van Tulder et al., 2003]. Centrally acting muscle relaxants are usually used in the treatment of neuropathic pain. Examples of these drugs; Gabapentin, Fosphenytoin, Tapentadol, Locasamide, Bicifadin. Fosphenytoin is a sodium channel blocker anticonvulsant showed significant analgesic effect in patients with central neuropathic pain following spinal cord injury compared to lignocain [Sang et al., 2006]. Tapentadol , a centrally acting analgesic acts by activation of *mu* opioid receptor and inhibit reuptake norepinephrine. Its analgesic potency is higher than corresponding tramadol but less than morphine [Tzchentke et al., 2006]. Carbamazepine is considered first-line therapy for trigeminal neuralgia. Clinical trials suggest its efficacy for treating diabetic neuropathy, but results are mixed for postherpetic neuralgia. Gabapentin is more effective than placebo at reducing diabetic neuropathy and postherpetic neuralgia-associated pain. In experimental animal model, inytrathecal gabapentin prevents the development of spinal opioid tolerance (Hansen et al., 2004]. Lamotrigine shows promise for decreasing pain associated with trigeminal neuralgia.

Baclofen

It is a derivative of γ-aminobutyric acid (GABA) primarily used to treat spasticity. It is a specific GABA-B receptor agonist and its beneficial effect results from actions at spinal and supraspinal sites unrelated to GABA. Tolerance does not seem to occur to any significant degree in that baclofen retains its therapeutic antispasmodic effects even after many years of chronic use [Gaillard, 1977]. Intrathecal baclofen is used for treatment moderate or severe generalized dystonia, particularly secondary dystonia [Albright et al., 2003]. Dykstra et al [2005] reported two cases with cervical dystonia who were not responded to oral medications and became resistant to botulinium toxin A and B injections but were successfully treated with high cervical (C1-C3) continuously infused (pump implant) intrathecal baclofen. Baclofen's site of action in treating dystonia is unknown. It may be at the spinal cord level or the cortical level or both. It is capable of inhibiting both monosynaptic reflexes at the spinal level, possibly by hyperpolarization of afferent terminals, although actions at supraspinal site may also occur and contribute to its clinical effects. The analgesic effect of baclofen may be related to inhibition of neural function presynaptically by reducing calcium ion influx and thereby reducing the release of excitatory neurotransmitters in both brain and spinal cord. Also it inhibits the release of substance P in the spinal cord [Cazalets et al., 1998].

Penerai et al [1985] found that baclofen pretreatment in human prolonged the duration of fentanyl-induced analgesia from 18 to 30 minutes in patients undergoing neurosurgical anesthesia.

Cyclobenzaprine

It is a tricyclic antidepressant compound that is used clinically as a long acting muscle relaxant and analgesic. It was originally shown to be of some benefit in the management of fibromyalgia in the mid-1980s [Lautenschlager, 2000]. It shares structural and pharmacological similarities with the tricyclic antidepressants [Rao, 2002]. Its mechanism of action may be mediated by blockade of 5-HT_2 receptors [Rao, 2002].

It was more effective than placebo for managing neck and back pain particularly in the first four days of therapy [Browning et al., 2001]. Cyclobenzaprine alone showed significant improvements in patients with acute neck and back pain with spasm but it did not showed significant synergistic effect with ibuprofen [Childers et al., 2005]

I. Biological Drugs

The clinical uses of these drugs are so limited in cervical spine disorders and they are still under experimental and clinical investigations. They are sub-grouped into:

1. Anti tumor necrosis factor-alpha (TNF_α)
2. Interleukin-1 (IL-1) blockers
3. Interleukin-1 (IL-1) Trap

1. Anti tumor necrosis factor-alpha (TNF_α) e.g. etanercept, infliximab, adalimumab, certolizumab.

Tumor necrosis factor-alpha (TNF_α) is a cytokine produced by monocytes and macrophages. It increases the migration of leucocytes to the inflammatory area. There are two types of TNF_α receptors found in leucocytes that respond to TNF by releasing other cytokines, and soluble TNF receptor that inactivate TNF and blunt the immune response.

Etanercept

It is a recombinant-DNA drug made by combining two proteins (a fusion protein). It links human soluble TNF-receptor to the Fc component of IgG_1. Etanercept mimics the inhibitory effects of naturally occurring soluble TNF receptor but has extended half-life in blood stream [Madhusudan et al., 2005]. It binds to TNF_α and decreases its role in disorders involving excess inflammation in humans and othe animals including autoimmune diseases such as ankylosing spondylitis [Braun et al., 2007], juvenile rheumatoid arthritis, psoriasis, psoriatic arthritis, rheumatoid arthritis. It was released for commercial use in late 1998. Experimental data showed that etanercept has a neurotoxic effect when injected into the endonerve [Wagner and Myers, 1996].

In controlled, non-randomized clinical study, patients with severe sciatica had sustained improvement, assessed by visual analogue scale for leg pain and for low back pain, after a short period of treatment with etanercept [Genevay and Singelin, 2004]. Zanella et al [2008] reported the significant long-lasting analgesic effect of a locally administered polymeric formulation of etanercept in an inflammatory neuropathic pain using unilateral chronic constriction injury of rat sciatic nerve. It did not affect the expression of CGRP neurons after nerve injury, therefore the analgesic effect of etanercept is not due to suppression of inflammatory neuropeptides [Norimoto et al., 2008]. Immediate intrathecal treatment with etanercept resulted in markedly reduced mechanical allodynia up to 4 weeks after spinal cord injury involved thoracic spinal cord hemisection [Marchand et al., 2008] This finding may offer therapeutic opportunities of etanercept for treating spinal cord injury pain.

2. Interleukin-1 (IL-1) Blockers
e.g. Anakinara

Interleukin-1 is a protein secreted by many cells in the body, it can trigger disease activity. Anakinara is an IL-1 receptor antagonist. It is recombinant, non glycosylated version of human IL-1 receptor antagonist. It is a biological response modifier. It is prepared from cultures of genetically modified *E. coli* using recombinant DNA technology. It blocks the biological activity of naturally occurring IL-1 including inflammation and cartilage degradation associated with rheumatoid arthritis by competitively inhibiting the binding of IL-1 to the IL-1 receptor which is expressed in many tissues and organs.

3. Interleukin-1 (IL-1) Trap
e.g. Rilonacept

Rilonacept prevents IL-1 from attaching to cell-surface receptors, creating a flare in disease. It was given as an orphan drug status by United States- Food and Drug administration. It is a dimeric fusion protein for the treatment of cryopyrin associated periodic syndromes including familial cold autoinflammatory syndrome and Muckle-Wells syndrome. Cryopyrin associated periodic syndrome associated syndrome is a life long, recurrent rash, fever, chills, joint pain, eye redness, eye pain and fatigue. These symptoms were triggered and exacerbated by cooling temperature, stress or exercise.

J. Adenosine

Endogenous denosine modulates the pain perception by activation the antinociceptive adenosine A_1-receptor within the central nervous system [Sawynok and Sweeney, 1989; Lee and Yaksh, 1998]. It is known that the antiallodynic effects of adenosine are mediated through the activation of spinal adenosine A_1 receptors and motor dysfunction effects are mediated through adenosine A_2 receptors at the spinal level [Lee and Yaksk, 1996]. Activation of adenosine A_1 receptors at the spinal level is required for the synergistic interaction on the mechanical allodynia [Park and Jun, 2008]. Spinally administered adenosine reduces hypersensitivity in animals and humans with nerve injury, but also causes transient pain in humans and reduces tonic inhibition in spinal neurons. In rats, intrathecal administration of ATP and the P2X-receptor agonist alpha, beta-methylene-ATP produced tactile allodynia which lasted more than 1 week and it is prevented by intrathecal administration of selective P2X3/P2X2/3 receptor antagonist [Nakagawa et al., 2007]. The antinociceptive effects of intrathecal adenosine were seen in a model of central neuropathic pain demonstrated in a model of spinal cord ischemia [Sjölund et al 1998]. Intrathecal injection of adenosine reduced the spontaneous and evoked pain in patients with chronic neuropathic pain [Belfrage et al., 1999]. Chronic intrathecal adenosine induces hypersensitivity in normal rats and that chronic blockade of spinal adenosine A_1 receptors by the A_1 antagonist 8-cyclopentyl-1,3-dipropylxanthine partially prevents nerve injury-induced hypersensitivity [Martin et al., 2006]. In human being chronic use of adenosine in a pump proved to be technically problematic and not advocated to use it [Lind et al., 2007].

K. Cholinergic Drugs

A major site of analgesic action of cholinergic agents is the spinal cord. Spinal cholinergic receptors have been shown to have a potent antinociceptive action. Activation of muscarinic acetylcholine receptor inhibits spinal nociceptive transmission by potentiation of GABAergic tone through M_2, M_3 and M_4 subtypes and increases the synaptic GABA release through calcium influx and voltage-gated calcium channels [Zhang et al., 2008]. It is believed that the analgesia after spinal cholinesterase inhibition by neostigmine is mediated through muscarinic, but not nicotinic cholinergic. Spinal administration of neostigmine produced a dose-dependent increase on the thermally evoked hind paw withdrawal latency in rats [Naguib and Yaksh, 1994]. Systemic administration of cholinesterase inhibitors which cross the blood brain barrier have long been known to produce analgesia and enhance analgesia from opiates. Spinal injection of cholinergic agonists results in analgesia to experimental, acute postoperative, and chronic pain which primarily reflects muscarinic receptor activation [Eisenach,1990]. In rats, both bethanechol and neostigmine reduced mechanical hyperalgesia [Prado and Dias, 2008].

L. Cannabinoids

Systemic or spinal administration of Δ^9-tetrahydrocannabinol (THC) and synthetic cannabinoids have antinociceptive and antihyperalgesic effects in a variety of animal models of acute and inflammatory pain [Pertwee, 2001; Iversen and Chapman, 2002]. The anti-nociceptive effects of THC or anandamide are mediated via CB_1-receptors (also known CNR1) and vanilloid (VR_1) receptor [DiMarzo et al., 2001]. THC and morphine potentiation was observed in tests of acute pain [Fuentes et al., 1999] and chronic inflammatory pain [Welch and Stevens, 1992]. There is evidence that supraspinal CB_2 (also known CNR2) receptors in the thalamus may contribute to the modulation of neuropathic pain responses [Jhaveri et al., 2008]. Cannabinoid agonists are already used clinically as antiemetic or to stimulate appetite. Potential therapeutic uses of cannabinoid receptor agonists include the management of multiple sclerosis, spinal cord injury, pain, inflammatory disorders, glaucoma, bronchial asthma and cancer [Singh and Budhiraja, 2006].

M. Non-Patch Type Topical Pain Relievers

Topical pain relieving drugs include preparations applied to the skin as cream, ointment, gel spray or patch. Topical drugs reduce the subcutaneous inflammation and soothe nerve pain. Topical analgesics differ from transdermal delivery systems, that is introduced in 1980, in that the latter's goal is to deliver systemic rather than local effects. Topical medicine used to treat pain associated with osteoarthritis, rheumatoid arthritis, neck or low back strain, whiplash, muscle inflammation and spasms and some types of nerve pain. The advantages of topical medicine include: its application is easy and controllable, the onset of symptoms relief is usually faster than oral preparations, also a steady rate and longer duration of symptom relief were observed with topical medicine,a smaller amount may be needed and topical medicine is not subjected to fast pass metabolism. The Disadvantages of topical medicine include certain types of back and neck pain will not respond to topical treatment and skin hypersensitivity reactions may occur. Topical analgesia include: Lidocaine (5%), Capsaicin (0.025-0.75%), Resiniferatoxin (0.00003-0.001%), Doxepin (3.3%), Amitriptyline (2%) and Ketamine (1%). They are effective moderately in peripheral neuropathic pain with allodynia and should consider as a therapeutic option but should be evaluated on an individual basis (Besson et al., 2008).

Ketamine

Lynche et al (2005a and b) demonstrated the effectiveness of 1% ketamine or 2% amitryptiline or 2% amitriptyline -1% ketamine combined in reducing the pain intensity assessed by 11 point numerical scale in neuropathic patients in randomized double blind placebo control and open labeled studies. In clinical reports, topical ketamine was reported to produce analgesia in case studies involving neuropathic and cancer pain [Crowley, 1998; Wood, 2000]. In experimental animal model ketamine produced an antihyperalgesic but not an analgesic action and produced no analgesia [Oatway et al., 2003]. Ketamine inhibits NMDA-receptors in neuronal preparations, and this could lead to the antihyperalgesic action [Hirota and Lambert 1996].

It is antihyperalgesic in acute inflammatory pain [Warncke et al., 1997] provides some direct analgesia [Pederson et al., 1998], inhibits sympathetically maintained pain [Crowley et al., 1998], but has no analgesic effects on capsaicin-induced hyperalgesia [Gottrup et al., 2000, 2004]

Amitriptyline

Ho et al (2008) found that 5% amitriptyline was ineffective in reducing pain intensity using a 0 to 100 mm visual analog scale in patients with neuropathic pain (postsurgical neuropathic pain, postherpetic neuralgia, or diabetic neuropathy with allodynia or hyperalgesia). There is evidence that trans-cutaneous amitriptyline solution has a differential effect on different fiber structures. It induced a mild and short-lasting increase of the tactile and mechanical nociceptive thresholds and it significantly decreased cold and heat thresholds [Dualé et al., 2008].

Amitriptyline produced both an antihyperalgesic and an analgesic action in the sensitized paw rat and produced analgesia in the nonsensitized paw rat [Oatway et al., 2003].

Amitriptyline like ketamine inhibits NMDA-receptors in neuronal preparations, and this could lead to the antihyperalgesic action [Reynolds and Miller, 1988].

Doxepin

Topical doxepin, a tricyclic antidepressant, produced analgesia in placebo-controlled trials of neuropathic pain [McCleane, 2000 a, b]. In the first study, doxepin (5%) was applied for 4 weeks, and produced significant analgesia in the last 10 days of treatment, but not in the 1st week. In the larger study, topical doxepin (3.3%) was compared with topical capsaicin (0.025%) and a combination of doxepin with capsaicin. Significant reductions in overall pain scores were observed for all treatment groups from week 2 to 4, but the combination group had a faster onset of action with analgesia at 1 week. A burning discomfort after cream application was noted by 81% in the capsaicin group, 61% in the doxepin/capsaicin group, and 17% in the doxepin group. Antidepressants exhibit promise as a useful class of agents to be used as analgesics following topical application and other methods of local delivery.

N. Spinal Injections

Intrathecal analgesia has emerged as a key therapeutic option for pain relief for patients who have failed other treatment avenues as well as patients with adequate analgesia on high dose entral or parentral therapy but with unacceptable side effects. Leonard Corning is credited with neuraxial administration of local anesthetic in 1885, and morphine may have been administered spinally as early as 1901[Matsuki, 1983].

Facet Joint Injection

The prevalence of facet joint pain is 55% in chronic cervical spinal pain [Manchikanti et al., 2004b]. Cervical facet pain is not characterized as easily as lumbar facet pain. It can occur with a variety of symptoms depending on the cervical level. Headache, neck pain spasm and general or focal neck pain can originate from the facet pain. This pain is typically worse when the patients extend or turn their neck. The upper cervical facets can often cause occipital headache. There are two methods of facet joint injection: the direct posterior and posterior-lateral approaches. A total amount of injected fluid is not usually more than 1.5 milliliter in the cervical spine (the capacity of a cervical facet joint is 0.5-1 milliliter). Common mixture is betamethasone, triamcinolone acetonide with bupivacaine, lidocaine. The optimal injection is made directly into the joint space. Pain relief following a precise intra-articular injection confirms the facet joint the source of pain. Long term relief (up to 6 months) can be obtained with steroids in 30-50% of patients. The most common causes that required facet joint injections are: degenerative disease, synovitis (overt or radiologically occult), post laminectomy syndrome and non radicular pain. Although facet joint injections rarely carried complications but they may include: bleeding, infection, allergic reactions, false negative response and accidental injection into vertebral artery or radicular branches can be dangerous. Some patients experience transient adverse effects (e.g. insomnia, nightmares) from the steroids and life-threatening idiopathic reaction to any medication was also observed. Facet joint injection is contraindicated in patients with history of allergy, coagulopathy, and severe foraminal stenosis because swelling of the joint may temporarily result in exacerbation of the patient's symptoms. Intra cervical zygapophyseal joints injections with the mixture of lidocaine [0.5 mL of 1%] and triamcinolone (5 mg) of patients with cervical zygapophyseal joint pain, were diagnosed originally as myofascial pain syndrome (MPS), cervical herniated nucleus pulposus (HNP), and whiplash-associated disorders (WAD) resulted in the immediate reduction of pain and the analgesic effect lasted longer in cervical HNP than MPS or WAD [Kim et al .,2005].

Selective Nerve Block, Transforaminal Epidural Injection

Epidural injections for managing chronic pain are one of the most commonly performed interventions in the United States [Manchikanti et al.,

2006]. Epidural steroid injections via a transforaminal approach, given the extremely small possibility for catastrophic complications that has been described. It is indicated in patients with radicular pain, with or without an axial component, originating from the cervical spine [Bush et al., 1996; Slipman et al., 2000]. It acts by suppression of the inflammatory response surrounding the targeted nerve roots [Molloy et al., 2005]. The complications of cervical transforaminal epidural steroid injection included acute infarction involving the cervical spine and extending to the cervicomedullary junction [Muro et al., 2007]. Scanlen et al [2007] demonstrated a significant risk (78 out of 1340 cases) of serious neurologic injury and mortality rate (~1%) after cervical transforaminal epidural steroid injections.

Intrathecal Pump

Morphine is the only opioid drug approved by the FDA for intreathecal delivary to treat chronic pain. Opioids administered neuraxially, act at receptors in the substantia gelatinosa of the spinal cord dorsal horn to yield dose-dependent analgesia [Pert and Snyder, 1973; Terenius, 1973]. Systemically administered morphine leads to an opioid-induced increase in spinal acetylcholine, and the opioid-induced spinal acetylcholine via activation of the spinal cholinergic system contributes to opioid-mediated antinociception [Nallu and Radhakrishnan, 2007]. Intrathecal (morphine) pump is used for chronic pain, cancer pain and for chronic spasticity. It increases pain relief in patients with severe pain and improves the quality of life and allows the patients to participate more fully in daily activities. A small pump is surgically placed under the skin of the abdomen to deliver medication directly into the area surrounded the spinal area via catheter. Long-term intrathecal opioid infusions can be effective in treatment of neuropathic pain but might require higher infusion doses [Anderson and Burchiel, 1999; Hassenbusch et al., 1995]. Hydromorphone, a semisynthetic hydrogenated ketone of morphine, is a more potent and faster-acting analgesic than morphine due to its greater lipophilic properties. Analgesic response was improved by a least 25% in patients with chronic nonmalignant pain who were switched from intraspinal morphine to hydromorphone because of poor pain relief [Anderson et al., 2001], and also the adverse reactions were improved. Intrathecal morphine and intrathecal hydromorphone (in a dose 20% of that of morphine) induce an equi-analgesic response [Ruan, 2007].

Sympathetic or Somatic Nerve Block

The occipital pain and headache of cervical arthritis also often respond to injection of 2 to 3 mL of long-acting anesthetic into the greater and lesser occipital nerves at the sites where they pierce the trapezius muscle [Carron, 1978].

Several drugs are currently used like steroids, local anaesthetics, opiods, muscle relaxants and α_2 adrenoceptor agonists.

Corticoteroids

It is believed that epidural administration of corticosteroids and/or local anesthetic altered or interrupted the nociceptive input, reflex mechanisms of the afferent fibers, self sustaining activity of the neurons, and the pattern of central neuronal activities. Corticosteroids reduce inflammation by inhibiting either the synthesis or release of a number of proinflammatory mediators and by causing a reversible local anaesthetic effect [Lundin et al., 2005; Lee et al., 1998]. Injections of corticosteroids into or adjacent to the spinal canal is performed on a regular basis in the United States. The use of methylprednisolone administration in the treatment of acute spinal cord injury is not proven as a standard of care, nor can it be considered a recommended treatment because its efficacy and impact is weak [John Hurlebert, 2000].

However, epidural steroids injections are used for herniated disc, sciatica, radiculopathy, spinal stenosis. Cervical epidural steroid injection have been used to treat the following conditions: pain associated with acute disc herniation and radiculopathy, postlaminectomy cervical pain, cervical strain syndromes with associated myofascial pain, and postherpetic neuralgia. Rowlingson and Kirschenbaum [1986] described significant reduction in upper extremity pain after cervical epidural steroid injections, and other studies identified radicular pain relief via interlaminar and transforaminal approaches. Transforaminal cervical epidural steroids injections provide long term pain relief in patients with neck pain and radiculopathy [Bush and Hillier, 1996] and cervical disc surgery [Lin et al., 2006; Kolstad et al., 2005]. The fact that corticosteroids differ significantly in microscopic size has become an important consideration because of an awareness that the larger a particle is, the greater are its chances of occluding a blood vessel should the compound be inadvertently injected vascularly. A study that analyzed the microscopic size of the aforementioned corticosteroids found the following:

Dexamethasone - Particles were 5-10 times smaller than red blood cells, contained few particles, and showed no aggregation.

Triamcinolone - Particles varied greatly in size, were densely packed, and formed extensive aggregations. It provides a sustained anti-inflammatory effect.

Betamethasone - Particles varied greatly in size, were densely packed, and formed extensive aggregations. It provides rapid onset and extended anti-inflammatory activity. The dose for intralaminar approach is 12-18 mg and half of this dose for transforaminal approach.

Methylprednisolone particles were relatively uniform in size, smaller than red blood cells, and densely packed and did not form very many aggregations. It provides a sustained anti-inflammatory effect. Because injected methylprednisolone has been reported to remain *in situ* for approximately 2 weeks, the clinician should expect to wait 2 weeks after the injection to assess the patient's response and to administer a repeat injection. The dose for intralaminar approach is 80-120 mg and half of this dose for transforaminal approach.

In cervical epidural injections, a total of 3-5 mL may be used for epidural steroid injections employing the interlaminar approach. However, in transforaminal approach, clinicians generally use a total volume of only about 1.5 mL. Neuraxial steroid injections are generally considered to be safe in the U.S. The following complications of steroid injections are reported:

(a) Direct spinal injury. Damage to the spinal cord at the level of the cervical spine will often result in greater impairment than will damage at the lumbar levels and may precipitate respiratory arrest at higher cervical levels. There is evidence that cervical epidural injection is rarely complicated by spinal cord injury and neurological deficit [Hodges et al., 1998; Brouwers et al., 2001]. The possible mechanism of injury is embolization of the spinal cord due to injection of steroid into a radicular artery Baker et al., 2003].
(b) Hematoma. Epidural hematoma occurs in 0.01-0.02% of performed procedures.
(c) Infection
(d) Inflammatory complications
(e) Others: anterior cord syndrome, presumably resulting from the injection of particulate into the artery of Adamkiewicz

Absolute contraindications for epidural steroid injections include the followings:

(a) Systemic infections or local infection at the site of a planned injection.
(b) Bleeding disorder or fully anticoagulated (for example, on a fully "therapeutic" dose of coumadin, heparin).
(c) History of significant allergic reactions to injected solutions (e.g. contrast, anesthetic, corticosteroids.
(d) Acute spinal cord compression
(e) Patient refusal to proceed with the injection procedure

Local Anaesthetics (Bupivacaine, Lidocaine)

Local anaesthetics interrupt the spine-spasm cycle and reverberating nociceptor transmission. Intrathecal local anesthetics are commonly used in combination with opioids. Intrathecal combinations of local anesthetics and opioids provided synergistic analgesic effects and decreased opioid side effects [van Dongen et al., 1999; Krames, 1993]. On the other hand a multicenter, double-blind randomized study found that the addition of bupivacaine did not provide better pain relief than opioids alone [Mironer et al., 2002].

Bupivaciane should not be used in place of lidocaine for needle procedures in the cervical spine. With inadvertent intrathecal injection, respiratory comprise may be prolonged due to bupivacaine's longer duration of action.

α_2 Adrenoceptor Agonists

α_2-adrenergic receptors play a key role in analgesic effects mediated at peripheral, spinal and brain stem sites. It hyperpolarizes the cell by increasing potassium conductance through G-protein (Gi) coupled K-channels on post synaptic neurons [Wallace andYaksh, 2000]. Also it activates spinal cholinergic neurons which may potentiate its analgesic effect. Clonidine is the only FDA-approved α_2-adrenoceptor agonist for intrathecal use. Intrathecal clonidine has been reported to provide significant analgesia alone or in combination with opioids for neuropathic pain, cancer pain, or complex regional pain syndrome [Ackerman et al., 2003; Uhle et al., 2000]. Siddall et al

[2000] assessed the efficacy of intrathecal morphine or clonidine, alone or combined for up to 6 days, in 15 patients with central pain secondary to spinal cord injury. They found the combination of clonidine and morphine provided significantly better pain relief than saline (37% *vs* 0% reduction) or either drug alone (20% reduction for morphine, 17% decrease for clonidine).

Ziconotide

It is the synthetic equivalent of ω-conopeptide MV1A, a 25-amino-acid polybasic peptide present in the venom of conus magus, a marine snail [Olivera et al., 1985]. It produces potent antinoceptive effect by selectively binding to N-type voltage-selective calcium channels [Olivera et al., 1987; Miljanich and Ramachandran, 1995] on neuronal soma, dendrites, dendritic shafts and axon terminals, thus blocking neurotransmission from primary nociceptive afferents. Intrathecal ziconotide provided clinically and statistically significant analgesia in patients with pain from cancer or acquired immune deficiency syndrome [Staats et al., 2004].

Baclofen

Baclofen is a GABA-B agonist that has been used for muscle spasms, spasticity, and neuropathic pain. Baclofen is a racemic mixture with L-baclofen being the active form.

Intrathecal baclofen infusions have been used to treat spasticity since the mid-1980s and intrathecal baclofen administration *via* an implanted device is approved by the Food and Drug Administration (FDA) for this indication. Intrathecal baclofen has been proven in reducing spasticity and dystonia associated with complex regional pain syndrome without any adverse effect [Taricco et al., 2006; van Hilten et al., 2000] but less effective in reducing neuropathic pain [Loubser and Akman, 1996].

Intrathecal Cocktails

Morphine sulfate combined with bupivacaine hydrochloride and clonidine hydrochloride incubated in implantable pumps at 37°C for 90 days remained stable with more than 96% of the original concentration intact. Combinations of morphine or hydromorphone with bupivacaine have been recognized to be stable [Hildebrand et al., 2001; Classen et al., 2004] but morphine and hydromorphone facilitate ziconotide degradation. A ziconotide/ clonidine/ morphine admixture was 70% stable for 20 days while Ziconotide/ baclofen admixtures are 80% stable over 30 days.

Chapter IV

Antimicrobials

Spinal infection can occur in vertebral bone, intervertebral disc space, epidural or intradural space within the spinal canal, and adjacent soft tissues. The most commonly isolated pathogen in 50% of bone infections is *Staphylococcus aureus* [Berbari et al., 2005]. Other microorganisms that have been implicated in bone infections include gram-positive microbes, such as *Streptococci* and *Enterococci*. Gram-negative bacteria such as *Enterobacteriaceae*, *Pseudomonas*, and anaerobic species are less frequently associated with bone infections [Lew and Waldvogel, 1997]. The pharmacokinetic characteristics of the antimicrobial molecule (including water or lipid soluble drug, molecular size, pH of drug, partition coefficient of drug, and protein binding) and the vascular integrity of bone are the most important factors that determined the drug bone penetration. Limited numbers of antimicrobials fulfill the above criteria and are useful in treatment of spinal infections.

Single dose of piperacillin-tazobactam produced concentrations in the cancellous and cortical bone that were sufficient to assure antibacterial activity [Incavo et al., 1994]. Successful treatment of cervical spinal epidural abscess was reported with piperacillin [Moriya et al., 2005]. Ticarcillin-clavulanate achieved high bone concentrations after a single 5.2 g bolus dose. Spontaneous pseudomonas osteomyelitis of spine was successfully managed with ticarcillin and tobramycin [Breit and Nade, 1987]. Ceftriaxone and cefamandole concentrations in the bone exceeded the minimum inhibitory concentration for susceptible staphylococcal pathogens [Lovering et al., 2001]. Similarly, cefazolin, a first-generation cephalosporin with excellent activity against *S. aureus*, was found to achieve bone tissue levels above minimum inhibitory concentrations for susceptible gram-positive organisms [Fass et al., 1978; Mader et al., 1989]. The mean synovial fluid concentration of cefoxitin obtained approximately half an hour after administration was >100% compared to the mean serum concentration obtained simultaneously [Schurman et al., 1982]. Meropenem effectively penetrated bone and joint tissue [Sano et al., 1993]. Rifampin is an effective adjunctive agent in treatment of staphylococcal infections. Cluzel et al [1984] reported that cancellous bone concentrations of rifampin were greater than the minimum inhibitory concentration of *S. aureus* strains up until 12 hours after a dose of 600 mg. Fluoroquinolones are attractive agents in the treatment of bone infections due to their broad antimicrobial activity and patient tolerability. A study investigating the penetration of levofloxacin into cortical and cancellous bone tissue and the synovial fluid concluded that the penetration as 100%, 50%, and 20% respectively [Rimmelé et al., 2004]. Single moxifloxacin dose 400 mg orally either 2 or 4 hours preoperatively achieved drug concentrations in the cancellous and cortical bone exceeding the minimum inhibitory concentrations for most pathogens [Malincarne et al., 2006]. Clindamycin has broad activity against gram-positive organisms such as streptococci and staphylococci and reasonably broad coverage of anaerobic bacteria. The concentration of clindamycin in infected bone was above the minimum inhibitory concentrations for susceptible *S. aureus* [Nicholas et al., 1975]. Metronidazole may be a useful adjunctive agent in polymicrobial bone infections. Its concentration in human bone is not well-defined. Macleod et al. [1986] investigated the penetration of aztreonam into synovial fluid and bone and found excellent tissue levels. Linezolid is a synthetic oxazolidinone antimicrobial agent with broad gram-positive activity including methicillin-resistant *Staphylococcus aureus* (MRSA) and methicillin-resistant *Staphylococcus epidermidis* (MRSE) [Bassetti et al., 2005]. The penetration of linezolid into bone was rapid, with a mean concentration of 9.1 mg/L 10 minutes after infusion 600 mg of the drug. The concentration of drug in the bone when compared with simultaneous blood concentrations was 51% at 10 minutes, 60% at 20 minutes, and 47% at 30 minutes [Lovering et al., 2002]. Linezolid concentration achieved in the tissue surrounding the bone was twice the minimum inhibitory concentration of the offending pathogens [Kutscha-Lissberg et al., 2003]. The vancomycin levels in bones were higher than the minimum inhibitory concentration for susceptible staphylococci following single prophylactic intravenous dose (15 mg/kg) [Graziani et al., 1988].

In spinal infections, antimicrobials are clinically indicated for discitis, osteomyelitis and epidural abscess.

Discitis

Discitis, an inflammation of the intervertebral disc, is generally attributable to *Staphylococcus aureus* and rarely *Staphylococcus epidermidis*, *Kingella kingae*, *Enterobacteriaciae*, and *Streptococcus pneumoniae*. Cervical discitis may be much more neurologically compromising due to anatomical particularities. Cottle and Riordan [2008] recommended that unless the patient is severely unwell antimicrobial therapy should be delayed until a microbiological diagnosis is established and tentative recommendations for antimicrobial therapy can be made based on theoretical considerations. It is still not known which antibiotics are able to penetrate the intervertebral disc effectively. Antibiotic use in discitis (in children) is controversial because the course of the disease appears to be benign [Cousins et al., 1992; Ryöppy et al., 1993; Wenger et al., 1978]. Ceftriaxone is recommended in children 3 years of age or younger because of the possibility of infection by *Haemophilus influenzae*. Postoperative disc space infection was prevented with a single prophylactic dose of a first-generation cephalosporin [Osti, 1990]. Tai et al. [2002] found that cefuroxime does not diffuse into human intervertebral discs as readily as gentamicin because the later is positively charged. There is considerable evidence to suggest that the charge on antibiotics, because of their ionisable groups, is important in determining their ability to diffuse into the disc [Rhoten et al., 1995; Scuderi et al., 1993]. In brief the following drugs penetrate the disc despite of their charge: cefazolin, ceftriaxone, cefuroxime, tobramycin, gentamycin, vancomycin ,teicoplanin and clindamycin. Natural or semisynthetic aminopenicillin not penetrate the intervertebral disc.

Brook [2001] reported two cases of septic discitis, one case due to *Peptostreptococcus magnus* treated with penicillin (intravenously) followed by oral ampicillin and the other showed fusiform Gram-negative bacilli with light growth *Fusobacterium nucleat*um treated with clindamycin. Vancomycin is effective against methicillin resistant staphylococcus aureus (MRSA) infections but it is less effective in treatment septic discitis due to MRSA [Al-Nammari et al., 2007]. In MRSA discitis animal model, vancomycin was superior to linezolid with a short treatment course [Conaughty et al., 2006]. The cure was achieved with long-term antimicrobial specific therapy with quinupristin-dalfopristin (50 days) and linezolid (100 days) in a case report with severe, chronic polymicrobial spine infection with epidural abscess and liquoral fistula due to multidrug-resistant organisms [Marroni et al., 2006]. A case report of cervical discitis, osteomyelitis, and epidural collection was cured with extended course of temocillin [Barton et al., 2008].

Spondylodiscitis with epidural abscess was reported to be successfully managed with ceftriaxone combined with cloxacillin [Lott-Duarte et al., 2008].

Pyogenic Osteomyleitis of the Cervical Spine

The large diameter of the cervical spinal cord relative to the spinal canal and the significant range of motion of the cervical spine make cervical osteomyelitis a unique entity. Hippocrates was the first to describe osteomyelitis of the spine in 400 BCE [cited from Dimar et al, 2004]. Establishing the diagnosis of cervical osteomyelitis in a timely fashion is critical to prevent catastrophic neurological injury [Dimar et al., 2004; Mc Henry et al., 2002]. Vertebral osteomyelitis of cervical spine accounts approximately 1-10% of all bone infections [Malawski and Lukawski, 1991; Schimmer et al., 2002]. The predominant organism in almost all studies is *Staphylococcus aureus,* accounting for approximately 40 to 80% of all spinal infections [Jensen et al., 1997]. Gram-positive organisms such as *S. epidermidis* and *Streptococcus* species are the second most common ones [Hadjipavlou et al., 2000]. Gram-negative bacteria such as *Escherichia coli*, *Diphtheroids*, *Pseudomonas, Salmonella* and *Proteus* species are also reported [Sapico et al., 1996] (Table 1). Polymicrobial infections and negative cultures are found in approximately 20% of patients [Sapico and Montgomerie, 1979, Sapico, 1996]. Blood cultures are positive in only approximately 20 to 60% of patients with spinal infection [Currier, 1998]. Mycobacterial or fungal infections should be considered in patients in whom results of cultures are persistently negative despite repeated tissue samples [Tandon and Vollmer, 2004]. Patients with overt signs of sepsis should be treated with intravenous broad-spectrum antibiotic drugs as soon as tissue is obtained for culture. Antibiotic therapy can then be tailored according to the culture and sensitivity results. Intravenous antibiotic drugs should be administered for 6 to 8 weeks, followed by a 6-week course of oral antibiotics until the infection is cured. Treatment with less than 4 weeks of antibiotic therapy is associated with a 25% relapse rate [Eismont et al., 1983; Sapico and Montgomerie, 1979; Sapico, 1996]. The erythrocyte sedimentation rate (ESR) can be expected to decrease to one half to two thirds of pretreatment levels on successful treatment [Sapico and Montgomerie, 1979; Sapico, 1996].

Epidural Abscess

Spinal epidural abscess has an estimated incidence rate of 0.2-2.8 cases per 10,000 per year with peak incidence occurring in people who are in their 60s and 70s. The most common causative agent is *staphylococcus aureus* [Martin and Yuan, 1996]. Spinal procedures (including spinal anesthesia, spinal surgery) or trauma, intravenous drug abuse, HIV infections, diabetes mellitus, alcoholism and malignancies are predisposing causes of spinal epidural abscess [Bartontini et al., 1996; Baker et al., 1975; Danner and Hartman, 1987]. The mainstay of treatment is surgical decompression. Non surgical treatment is indicated in patients with minimal neurological deficit or are poor surgical candidates [Manfredi et al., 1998]. High doses cefazolin/clindamycin combination is highly effective for patients with epidural abscess [de Goeij et al., 2008; Solomou et al., 2004; Walters et al., 2006].

Chapter V

Complementary/Alternative Analgesia

Complementary/alternative medicine (CAM) has been defined as, "diagnosis, treatment and/or prevention that complements mainstream medicine by contributing to a common whole, by satisfying a demand not met by orthodoxy or by diversifying the conceptual frameworks of medicine [Ernst et al., 2001].

Many different CAM modalities are used to treat pain; amongst the most popular are:

Acupuncture
Trigger points
Mind-body therapy
Magnet therapy
Prolotherapy
Exercise
Spinal manipulation
Herbal preparations
Nutritional supplements

Acupuncture

It is believed that the analgesic effect of acupuncture is related to the stimulation of endorphins, serotonin, and noradrenaline secretion in the central nervous system, or release of vasodilators such as histamine (which modulate the vascular tone) or closing the gates of nerve fibers that result in pain perception. Conflicting results were reported about the effectiveness of acupuncture in neck pain. The outcomes of 14 randomized controlled trials were equally balanced between positive and negative. Acupuncture was superior to waiting-list in one study, and either equal or superior to physiotherapy in three studies, it was not superior to indistinguishable sham control in four out of five studies and five out eight high-quality trials were negative [White and Ernst,1999]. There is evidence that acupuncture needles placed in non acupuncture points lead to pain reduction because of stimulation of endorphin release *via* a mechanism called diffuse noxious inhibitory control [LeBars et al., 1979]. Acupuncture and other forms of acustimulation are effective in the short-term management of neck pain [Wang et al., 2008]. The success rate was higher in patients with a short duration of chronic neck pain [Blossfeldt, 2004]. Acupuncture may facilitate and/or enhance physiotherapy performance in musculoskeletal rehabilitation for tension neck syndrome in term of improving pain intensity, muscle tension, the neck disability index, and the cranio-cervical flexion test for isometric neck muscle strength [França et al., 2008]. The efficacy of acupuncture is approximated that of 0.5% lidocaine injection of trigger points in improving pain scores, range of neck movement, pressure pain intensity and depression in elderly patients with myofascial pain syndrome [Ga et al., 2007]. Trigger point acupuncture compared with standard acupuncture is significantly reduced the pain intensity and improved quality of life in patients with non radiated chronic neck pain with normal neurological examination [Itoh et al., 2007]. Guo et al [2007] found that abdominal acupuncture can significantly reduce the neck pain of the patient caused by cervical spondylosis as the traditional acupuncture.

Trigger Points

They are discrete, hyperirritable foci usually located within a taut band of skeletal muscle [Simons et al., 2002]. Pressure applied to these points produce a characteristic referred pain, tenderness and autonomic phenomena. They are an essential defining part of the myofascial pain syndrome, in which widespread or regional muscular pain is a cause of musculoskeletal dysfunction [Gerwin, 2002]. Trigger points are reported to occur more frequently in cases of mechanical neck pain than in matched controls [de Las Penas et al., 2007]. There are two types of trigger points; active and lantent.

Active trigger point that defined as one with spontaneous pain, or pain in response to movement. It is tender on palpation, and may present with a referral pattern of pain, not at the site of the trigger point origin e.g. fibromyalgia [Simons, 1986] and neck pain [Sist et al., 1999]. Rosomoff's team demonstrated that 100% of neck pain sufferers possessed the presence of trigger points and almost 53% of them had non-dermatomal referral [Rosomoff et al., 1989]. Latent trigger point is a sensitive spot that causes pain or discomfort only in response to compression. The pathogenesis of trigger points may be due to decrease in the pain pressure threshold [Fischer, 1986], or release of inflammatory mediators e.g. prostaglandins, bradykinin, serotonin or trauma [Alvarez and Rockwell, 2002]. Manual therapy [Hong et al., 1993], chiropractic treatment [Hsieh and Hong, 1990], electric therapy [Hsueh et al., 1997], local anaesthetic [McMillan et al., 1997] and active therapy [Hanten et al., 2000] have all been claimed to provide relief of trigger point sensitivity.

It is postulated that massage and myofascial release aim to increase local circulation, improve mobility and relieve subcutaneous tightness. Neuro Emotional Technique (NET) was administered to provide participants with a mind/body based treatment to relieve the sensitivity of trigger points associated with their chronic neck pain.

This technique significantly relieved pain sensitivity of trigger points presenting in a a cohort of chronic neck pain sufferers [Bablis et al., 2008]. The visual analog scale significantly decreased in sensitivity as well as pressure algometer readings significantly increased after a single NET treatment.

Mind-Body Therapy

It is behavioral, psychological, social, and spiritual approaches to medicine not commonly used. It includes: mediation, imagery, biofeedback, relaxation and hypnosis. This therapy may be effective in patients who have had rheumatoid arthritis for a short time [Astin et al., 2002]. Mindfulness meditation may be an effective strategy for helping chronic pain patients who cope more effectively with their conditions [Kabat-Zinn et al., 1985, 1987].

Magnet Therapy

Magnets may also be perceived as a more natural and less harmful alternative to analgesic compounds. It involves the application of magnetic materials on or very close to the skin over prolonged periods of time. This encompasses a wide range of interventions involving different types of devices, different strength magnetic fields and different modes of administration [Hinman, 2002]. Magnet therapy now appears to be one of the most widely used form of CAM for the management of chronic pain associated with musculoskeletal disorders such as rheumatoid arthritis. Despite the popularity of using magnets for healing pain, there is a lack of scientific evidence to prove magnets have any therapeutic benefit. Several theories were claimed, not scientifically supported, the mechanism of magnet therapy for pain heeling. These are:

1. Restoration of cellular magnetic balance.
2. Migration of calcium ions is accelerated to help heal bones and nerve tissues.
3. Circulation is enhanced since biomagnets are attracted to the iron in blood and this increase in blood flow helps healing.
4. Biomagnets have a positive effect on the pH balance of cells.
5. Hormone production is influenced by biomagnet use.

Several studies described the site, magnet support device and frequency and duration of static magnetic field (SMF) therapy but most studies failed to provide enough detail about SMF dosage to permit protocol replication by other investigators [Colbert et al., 2007].

Prolotherapy or Proliferative Injection Therapy or Regenerative Injection Therapy

Historically, the use of prolotherapy dates back to Hippocrates who treated dislocated shoulders of soldiers on the battlefields with red-hot needle cautery to stabilize the joint.

Hackett defined prolotherapy as "the rehabilitation of an incompetent structure [ligament or tendon] by the generation of new cellular tissue," and concluded that "a joint is only as strong as its weakest ligament"[Hackett et al., 1992]. Prolotherapy is a method of injection treatment designed to stimulate healing. It involves injecting an otherwise non-pharmacological and non-active irritant solution into the body, generally in the region of tendons or ligaments for the purpose of strengthening weakened connective tissue and alleviating musculoskeletal pain. This treatment is used for musculoskeletal pain which has gone on longer than 8 weeks such as low back and neck pain, chronic sprains and/or strains, whiplash injuries, tennis and golfer's elbow, knee, ankle, shoulder or other joint pain, chronic tendonitis/ tendonosis, and musculoskeletal pain related to osteoarthritis. It is based on the premise that chronic musculoskeletal pain is due to inadequate repair of fibrous connective tissue, resulting in ligament and tendon weakness or laxity [Leadbetter, 1994; Frank et al., 1985]. The injection is given into joint capsules or where tendon connects to bone. Many points may require injections. The Injected solution causes the body to heal itself through the process of inflammation and repair. Prolotherapy treatment sessions are generally given every two to six weeks. Many solutions are used, including dextrose, lidocaine (a commonly used local anesthetic) procaine, phenol (an alcohol), glycerine, or cod liver oil extract. The most common proliferant used in prolotherapy injections is hypertonic dextrose, 12.5% to 25%, with 15% being the most used. Once the cell fluid is able to dilute the dextrose, the inflammation ceases but growth factor activation continues [Reeves, 1995].

Local injection causes temporary, low grade inflammation at the site of ligament or tendon weakness (fibroosseous junction) leads to migration and activation the fibroblasts which synthesize precursors to mature collagen, and thereby reinforcing connective tissue [Reeves, 2000]. This inflammatory stimulus raises the level of growth factors to resume or initiate a new connective tissue repair sequence to complete one which had prematurely aborted or never started. Hackett reported that 82% of patients with low back pain, treated with dextrose or saline injections, considered themselves cured over periods ranging up to 12 years of follow-up [Hackett, 1959]. A series of injections of dextrose solution injected into the neck improved pain symptoms and quality of life in chronic neck pain suffers [Hauser and Hauser, 2007]. Intraarticular regeneration injection therapy improved pain and function in patients with chronic whiplash related neck pain that failed other conservative and interventional procedures [Hooper et al., 2007]. Patients were treated with intraarticular prolotherapy by placing 0.5 - 1mL of 20% dextrose solution (D50W with 1% lidocaine) into each zygapophysial joint. Dagenais et al [2007] reviewed high quality studies with a total of 366 participants with chronic low-back pain managed with prolotherapy and other co-interventions and found that prolotherapy alone was not effective therapy but may improve pain when it combined with spinal manipulation, exercise, and other co-interventions. Over 99 percent of 10,000 prolotherapy cases, found relief from their chronic pain [Hauser, 1999]. Prolotherapy is contraindicated in infections, immunodeficiency conditions, acute gout, rheumatoid arthritis, cervical stenosis, and current use of narcotics, steroids and nonsteroidal anti-inflammatory drugs. The most common risk of such therapy is bruising around the injected area. Pain after treatment, infection, and allergy are also reported.

Exercise

Exercise interventions are deemed for the effective management of patients with neck pain. Janda [1994] suggested that the cervical flexor muscles become dysfunctional in the presence of neck pain. When exercise planed for treatment, it is necessary to have an understanding of abnormalities in the muscular system associated with painful dysfunctional joints. Two types of exercise programs, based on the muscle deficits considered to occur in neck pain, have been proposed to address cervical flexor muscle impairment. The first exercise regime consists of general strengthening and endurance excercises for the neck flexor muscles [Jordan et al., 1998; Bronfort et al., 2001]. These exercises involve high load training and they recruit all the muscle synergists that is, both the deep and superficial muscles. This program trained the cervical flexors muscles with the controlled head lift exercise and focus on training endurance and increasing the number of repetitions [Berg et al., 1994, Bronfort et al., 2001].

The second exercise regime has been designed to focus on the muscle control aspects and aims at improving control of the muscles within the neck flexor synergy (Jull et al 2004].

Specific exercise program significantly reduced the frequency of headache and neck pain and results were maintained in the long term at the 12 month follow-up.

Spinal Manipulation

The American Chiropractic Association [2007] defines spinal manipulation as a passive manual maneuver "during which the three joint complex may be carried beyond the normal voluntary physiological range of movement into the para-physiologic space without exceeding the boundaries of anatomic integrity. Most of spinal manipulation studies focus on low back pain which showed it was not superior to pharmacological interventions [Assendelft et al., 2003].

The mechanisms responsible for the effective pain relief and restoration of functional ability documented after spinal manipulation of dysfunctional cervical joints may be due to alteration in specific central corticomotor facilitatory and inhibitory neural processing and cortical motor control of upper limb muscles in a muscle-specific manner [Taylor and Murphy, 2008].

One study showed that C7-T1 spinal manipulation improved the pain pressure threshold in health individuals without a current history of neck pain in C5-C6 zygapophyseal joints [de-Las-Peñas et al., 2008]. Spinal manipulation, if not contraindicated, may be the only treatment modality of the assessed regimens that provides broad and significant long-term benefit compared with acupuncture or medications [Muller and Giles, 2005]. Data of three randomized controlled trials consisted of 329 patients with non-specific neck pain in an adult (18-70years) showed that up to 25% clinically relevant improvement in pain [Schellingerhout et al., 2008].

Nutraceuticals

The recent recommendations of American College of Rheumatology (ACR) guidelines for treating OA [2000] included dietary supplements, such as glucosamine sulfate, chondroitin sulfate, and antioxidants, as well as acupuncture and magnets as therapies under investigation.

Glucosamine

Glucosamine is an amino sugar and a prominent precursor in the biochemical synthesis of glycosylated proteins and lipids. Since glucosamine is a precursor for glycosaminoglycans, and glycosaminoglycans are a major component of joint cartilage, supplemental glucosamine may help to rebuild cartilage and treat arthritis. In the United States, glucosamine is not approved by the Food and Drug Administration for medical use in humans. It has the following pharmacological actions:

(a) Antiinflammatory [Largo et al., 2003;Chan et al., 2006]
(b) Stimulates the synthesis of proteoglycans [Bassleer et al., 1998]
(c) Reduces the catabolic activity of chondrocytes by inhibiting the synthesis of proteolytic enzymes and other substances that contribute to damage cartilage matrix [Dodge and Jimenez, 2003; Chan et al., 2005]

There have been multiple clinical trials of glucosamine as a medical therapy for osteoarthritis, but results have been conflicting. Reginster et al [2001] and Pavelka et al [2002] showed a clear benefit for glucosamine treatment while Hughes and Carr [2002] and Cibere et al [2004] did not detect any benefit of glucosamine. Some reviews and meta-analyses have evaluated the efficacy of glucosamine. Richy et al [2003] performed a meta-analysis of randomized clinical trials in 2003 and found glucosamine efficacy on VAS and Western Ontario MacMaster Questionnaire (WOMAC) pain, Lequesne index and visual analog scales (VAS) mobility and good tolerability. Recently, a review by Bruyere and Reginster [2007] about glucosamine and chondroitin sulfate for the treatment of knee and hip osteoarthritis concluded that both products act as valuable symptomatic therapies for osteoarthritis disease with some potential structure-modifying effects. OsteoArthritis Research Society International (OARSI) is recommending glucosamine as the second most effective treatment for moderate cases of osteoarthritis.In vitro, experimental study of interleukin-1 (IL-1) stimulated rat, glucosamine completely inhibited IL-6 and TNF-alpha and increased nitric oxide with no effect to annulus cells viability [Walsh et al., 2007].

Chondroitin Sulfate

It is a sulfated glycosaminoglycan composed of a chain of alternating sugars (N-acetylgalactosamine and glucuronic acid). It is usually found attached to proteins as part of a proteoglycan. Chondroitin sulfate is an important structural component of cartilage and provides much of its resistance to compression. It is approved and regulated as a symptomatic slow-acting drug for osteoarthritis in Europe and some other countries [Jordan and Arden, 2003].

Methylsulfonylmethane

It is an organosulfur compound with colorless solid. It occurs naturally in some primitive plants and is present in small amounts in many foods and beverages. Usha and Naidu [2004] found that 1500 mg per day methylsulfonylmethane (alone or in combination with glucosamine sulfate) was helpful in relieving symptoms of knee osteoarthritis. Moreover, Kim et al [2006] reported that patients, with osteoarthritis of knee, treated with methylsulfonylmethane for several weeks had significantly reduced pain and improved physical functioning, without major adverse events.

Avocado-Soybean Unsaponifiables

This preparation was superior in both pain control and functional measures in patients with osteoarthritis [Ernst, 2003].

Omega-3- Fatty Acids

Fish oil is rich in omega-3-fatty acids have antiinflammatory activity through their effects on prostaglandin metabolism. Several randomized controlled trials have shown clinical benefit of fish oil supplementation in rheumatoid arthritis [McCarthy and Kenny, 1992].

S-Adenosyl Methionine

It is one of the dietary supplements that gained popularity, and was recently reported to be effective in the management of depression, liver disease and arthritis. It is produced endogenously from methionine and adenosine triphosphate (ATP). It is an important methyl group donor playing an essential role in many biochemical reactions involving enzymatic transmethylation that play an important role in the biosynthesis of phospholipids that are important for the integrity of cell membranes. In *in vitro* studies using human articular chondrocytes have shown SAMe-induced increases in proteoglycan synthesis [Harmand et al., 1987] and proliferation rates in rabbits [Barcelo et al., 1987].

SAMe may reduce inflammatory mediators thus reducing pain. This was noted in other studies with the reduction of TNF-α and fibronectin RNA expression using cultured rabbit synovial cells [Gutierrez et al., 1997]. SAMe has a slower onset of action but is as effective as celecoxib in the management of symptoms of knee osteoarthritis [Najm et al., 2004]. It improves, possibly through analgesic and anti-inflammatory properties, the disease activity, pain, fatigue, morning stiffness and mood of patients with fibromyalgia [Jacobson et al., 1991].

In brief, potential mechanisms of nutraceuticals in osteoarthritis include:

(a) Increase the synthesis of glycosaminoglycan , prostaglandins and hyaluronic acid
(b) Increase synthesis of aggrecan
(c) Inhibit metalloproteinase involved in cartilage breakdown.
(d) Inhibit IL-1 induced increases aggercanases activity
(e) Inhibit nitric oxide production induced by IL-1 and TNF

Herbal Medicines

The most popular forms of complementary treatments are herbal medicines. In the United States, the annual expenditure on herbal remedies exceeds 1.5 billion dollars and grows each year by approximately 25% [Muller and Clauson, 1997]. Most of the herbal medicines have an effect on the eicosanoid metabolism, inhibiting one or both of the cyclooxygenase and lipoxygenase pathways. Ideal extract doses and treatment periods still have to be determined. In most cases, herbal treatments are based on traditional use, which is a notoriously unreliable indicator of effectiveness [Ernst, 1998]. Herbal medicines are advantageous because they do not have dangerous adverse reactions that occurred from long-term use of steroids or non steroidal anti-inflammatory drugs. The following herbs are traditionally used as analgesics:

Cayenne (Capsicum Frutescens)

The active ingredient of cayenne is capsaicin. Patients with fibromyalgia receiving the active therapy (capsaicin plasters) experienced less tenderness and significant increase in grip strength [McCarthy et al., 1994; Gagnier et al., 2007].

St John's Wort (Hypericum Perforatum)

It affects nerve and is effective for sharp, shooting nerve pains. In laboratory animals, Hypericum perforatum extract shows significant antinociceptive effect and it potentiates morphine induced antinociceptive effect [Uchida et al., 2008].

Siberian Gingseng

It resolves the fatigue associated with fibromyalgia.

Tumeric

It reduces pain and inflammation. Curcumin is the active compound in tumeric. Curcumin is effective as cortisone and phenylbutazone in decreasing inflammation. It blocks the effect of substance P on neuron besides it reduces the levels of prostaglandins, TNF-alpha and nitric oxide [Sharma et al., 2007].

Calendula Officinalis
(Also Known as Marigold)

In Italian folk medicine calendula is used as an antipyretic and anti-inflammatory. It is used to revere symptoms of fibromyalgia. Recently it is studied in combination with other natural product, as direct anticytokine therapy with maximum anti-inflammatory on cell model of inflammation [Gorchakova et al., 2007].

Devil's Claw Root (Harpagophytum Procumbens)

It is a natural anti-inflammatory used to treat rheumatic disorders. The herbal preparation was reported as significantly better than placebo for pain reduction and increased the mobility in patients with osteoarthritis [Guyader, 1984; Lecomte and Costa, 1992].

Willow Bark (Salix Alba)

It contains a chemical similar to aspirin. The active ingredient is salicin which is transformed in the stomach to salicylic acid. Willow bark extracts have analgesic, antiinflammatory and antipyretic effects and therefore may be important in treatment of neck pain. There is evidence that willow bark has short term improvement in pain of spine [Gagnier et al., 2007].

Feverfew (Tanacetum Parthenium)
Sometimes Called a "Summer Daisy

It has analgesic and anti-inflammatory properties due to reducing the prostaglandins production. The active ingredient is parthenolide that inhibits the prostaglandins production but it does not inhibit cyclooxygenases [Kwok et al., 2001]. Parthenolide also specifically binds to and inhibits IκB kinase complex (IKK)β, an important proinflammatory cytokine [Collier et al.,1980; Brown et al., 1997].

Dong Quai (Radix Angelicae sinesis)

Also known as Chinese angalica, female ginseng It is good for fleeting muscle and joint pains. Dong quai is traditionally used in the treatment of arthritis. However, there is insufficient reliable human evidence to recommend the use of Dong quai alone or in combination with other herbs for osteoarthritis or rheumatoid arthritis.

Licorice (Glycyrrhiza Glabra) Root

It acts in the body like cortisone. Licorice, ginseng, bupleurum stimulate the pituitary and adrenal glands to increase natural production of cortisone [Wu, 2008].Because licorice can affect the metabolism of steroids, licorice is sometimes used to decrease inflammation.

Dandelion (Taraxacum Officinale)

It reduces frequency and intensity of pain and strength the connective tissue. In laboratory animals dandelion root may possess anti-inflammatory properties but there is a lack of well-conducted human studies in this area.

Ginger (Zingiber Officinale) Tea

It is good alternative to aspirin to relieve minor aches and pains. It has long been used in India to treat inflammation and pain. It relieves the pain of muscle spasm, rheumatoid arthritis and osteoarthritis by lowering prostaglandins level [Frondoza et al., 2004; Shen et al., 2005; Lantz et al., 2007]

Pomegrante(Punica Granatum L.)

Extracts of pomegranate fruit have been shown to possess anti-inflammatory and cartilage sparing effects *in vitro* [Ahmed et al., 2005]. It has been shown that pomegranate extract exerted a powerful influence in inhibiting the expression of inflammatory cytokines IL-1and IL-6 in adjunctive periodontal therapy [Sastravaha et al., 2005]. Shukla et al [2008] found that pomegranate extract inhibits the IL-1-induced PGE2 and NO production in rabbit chondrocytes, and also inhibits both COX-1 and COX-2 enzyme activity *ex vivo* but the effect was more pronounced on the enzyme activity of COX-2 enzyme.

Gamma-Linolenic Acid (GLA)-Containing Herbs

Blackcurrant (*Ribes nigrum*) seeds contain high levels of GLA, an essential fatty acid that exerts anti-inflammatory activity by interfering with prostaglandin metabolism [Darlington and Stone, 2001]. It suppresses the release of inflammatory mediators, perhaps by direct effect on T cell. It showed significant reduction in pain as compared with placebo in patients with rheumatoid arthritis. In one randomized controlled study, blackcurrant seed oil did not show objective signs of reduced activity of rheumatoid arthritis [Levanthal et al., 1994].

Ayurvedic preparation

Ayurvedic medicine is an ancient system of healing that originated in India over 4000 years ago. Ayurvedic preparation, has demonstrated anti-inflammatory activity in vitro by reducing leukotriene synthesis [Ammon et al., 1993].

Pine-bark extract: it is natural anti-inflammatory
Grape seeds extract: it is natural anti-inflammatory

Moreover, topical application of Cayenne (Capsicum) mixed with wintergreen oil can help to relieve muscle pain and the following mixture of passion flower, valerian hops tea have sedative and muscle relaxant properties. *Phytodolor* is a standardised herbal preparation of *Populus tremula, Fraxinus excelsior* and *Solidago virgaurea* (ratio 3:1:1) used for the treatment of musculoskeletal pain. It may have anti-inflammatory properties, and it is thought to inhibit arachidonic acid metabolism via the cyclooxygenase and lipoxygenase pathways, leading to suppression of inflammation. Significant pain relief and joint mobility was observed in rheumatoid patients received this herbal preparation [Ernst and Chrubasik, 2000; Ernst, 1999].

Certain active ingredients are extracted from herbs and plants are used as analgesics. Examples of these substances are quercetin and bromelain. *Quercetin* is a flavonol. It found in capers, lovage, apples, tea, onion espicially red onion, red grapes, citrus fruit, tomato, leafy green vegetables and in varieties of honey. Quercetin has demonstrated significant anti-inflammatory activity because of direct inhibition of several initial processes of inflammation including inhibition of inflammatory leukotriene production. It inhibits both the synthesis and release of histamine and other allergic/ inflammatory mediators. In addition, it exerts potent antioxidant and antitumor properties [Paliwal et al., 2005]. Experimentally, it inhibits uric acid production in a manner similar to allopurinol, as well as inhibits synthesis and release of inflammatory compounds. In animals Quercetin induces an antinociceptive effect and when combined with clonidine produces a synergistic analgesic effect [Kaur et al., 2005]. *Bromelain* is an enzyme from the stem of the pine apple, inhibits prostaglandins production and reduces the inflammation due to arthritis or sport injury [Klein and Kullich, 1999]. It is currently used for pain relief in a number of US hospitals.

Chapter VI

Quality of Life

There is no doubt that neck pain can influence the patient's quality of life. There are several instruments for assessment the quality of life (QoL) in patients with pain.

Kovacs et al [2008] compared the psychometric characteristic of the Spanish version of the Northwick Pain Questionnaire with Neck Disability Index Questionnaire (NDI), and the Core Outcome Measure (COM) in patients with nonspecific chronic pain. The authors found that neck disability index seems to be the best instrument for measuring neck pain-related disability because the core outcome measure and Northwick pain questionnaire are worse and its use may lead to patients' evolution seeming more positive than it actually is.

Forestier et al [2007] suggested the Copenhagen Neck Functional Disability Scale (CNFDS) as a good tool for evaluating neck pain because its scores were normally distributed and were less sensitive to change than the visual analogue scale pain scores, the short-form-36 quality-of-life instrument (SF-36), and more sensitive to change than the other efficacy criteria. Individuals seeking care for neck or back pain have worse health status [assessed by health related quality of life and pain intensity] than those who do not seek care [Côté et al., 2001]. Health-related quality of life as measured by the SF-36 Short Form questionnaire is strongly affected by orofacial pain [Kohlmann, 2002]. Even controlling for gender, age, and number of pains during the past 7 days statistically significant reduction of scores in 5 out of 6 SF-36 subscales was observed in those with prevalent orofacial pain. Long term neck pain may influence the quality of life. Wallin and Raak [2008] evaluate the health related quality of life in whiplash associated disorder

(WAD) patients using the SF-36 and found WAD patients are scored lower on the SF-36 in all scales when compared with healthy pain-free individuals. According to Bono et al data [2000] who used the short form Health Survey (SF-36), whiplash patients showed an impairment of cervical spine mobility, as well as a poor QoL, compared to a control group population

Rezai et al [2008] examined the association between grades of neck pain and, physical and mental components of health related –quality of life (HR-QOL) using SF-36 health survey. Their results showed that individuals with chronic neck pain with grade III-IV had significant lower physical and mental components, and the author attributed these findings to co-morbidities. Both standard physical therapy (including hot pack, ultrasound therapy and exercise program) traction therapy in addition to standard physical therapy improved significantly in pain intensity, the scores of neck disability index and physical subscales of quality of life assessed by Nottingham Health Profile in patients with nonspecific chronic pain [Borman et al., 2008].

Certain assessment of patients with neck pain may optimize the efficacy of rehabilitation program. Börsbo et al [2008] assessed 275 consecutive chronic pain patients with whiplash associated disorders using self-report questionnaires related to pain intensity in neck and shoulders, Beck Depression Inventory, Catastrophizing scale of coping strategy questionnaire, life satisfaction checklist, the SF-36 health survey and EurQoL. The authors found that the degree of depression appears to be the most important influencing factor to perceived health and quality of life in patients with whiplash-associated disorders. Haines et al [2008] assessed patient education strategies for neck pain at three advices focusing on activation, pain and stress coping skills and "traditional neck school" and found ineffective educational interventions in various disorder types and follow-up periods. EuroQol (EQ-5D) had the highest overall ability to predict return to work or not return to work irrespective of gender, neck or low back pain or duration of the problems in cohort of 1,575 men and women sick-listed more than 28 days due to back or neck problems [Hansson et al., 2006.] In a cross-sectional study was conducted on 2356 patients with neck pain, 171 of them who received worker's compensation showed significant lower SF-36 scores for Physical Functioning [Hee et al., 2002] Trigger point acupuncture therapy is more effective than aqupoints or non-trigger point acupuncture in reducing pain intensity and improving the quality of life in aged patients with chronic neck pain [Itoh et al., 2007]. Pulsed radiofrequency treatment of the cervical dorsal root ganglion may provide pain relief for limited number patients with chronic cervical radicular pain for a mean period of 9.2 months and significantly improved the quality of life in the SF-36 domain vitality at 3 months. There were no important differences in quality-adjusted life expectancy associated with standard non steroidal anti-inflammatory drugs, selective COX-2 inhibitors, exercise, mobilization, and manipulation in patients with nonspecific chronic pain [van der Velde et al., 2008]. Ma et al [2007] found that oxycondone controlled release could be an important optional drug for the management of refractory and frequent acute episodes of chronic neck pain, it improves the pain, sleep and quality of life as the most domains of SF-36 were improved. Neck pain had a significant impact on all SF-36 domains and represented the main determinant of depression in cervical dystonia. Botulinium neurotoxin type (A) therapy resulted in a significant improvement of clinical symptoms in cervical dystonia and only two of the eight SF-36 domains improved significantly in patients with cervical dystonia [Müller et al., 2002]. Botulinum neurotoxin type (A) treatment has some efficacy when administered within 1 year of the whiplash injury and improves the quality of life as evaluated by the SF-36 questionnaire but it does not reach to the significant level [Braker et al., 2008]. Cano et al [2006] found that the Subscales of the cervical dystonia impact profile (CDIP-58) were more sensitive in detecting statistical and clinical change than comparable subscales of the Medical Outcome Study Short Form-Health Survey (SF-36), Functional Disability Questionnaire (FDQ), and Toronto Western Spasmodic Torticollis Rating Scale (TWSTRS) in patients with cervical dystonia treated with botulinum toxin (A).

Conclusion

The above review has focused on specific targets and classes of drugs that are used in management of neck pain. In recognizing the complexity of causes of neck pain, it is important to take in consideration that the optimal pain relief may require combinations of more than one agent, more than one pharmaceutical preparation and sometimes spinal injections. With certain conditions like cephalogenic headache and fibromyalgia , combinations could include any number of multiple targets for pain mediators while with cervical dystonia , neurotoxins could resole the problem. Tolerance and dependence may occur in patients with chronic pain then alternative strategies may combat them. Traditional medicines play a role in management of neck pain and antimicrobials should be appropriately selected in treatment of spinal infections.

References

Ackerman, LL; Follett, KA; Rosenquist, RW. Long-term outcomes during treatment of chronic pain with intrathecal clonidine or clonidine/opioid combinations. *J Pain Symptom Manage,* 2003, 26, 668-677.

Agarwal, S; Polydefkis, M; Block, B; Haythornthwaite, J; Raja, SN. Transdermal fentanyl reduces pain and improves functional activity in neuropathic pain states. *Pain Med,* 2007, 8, 554-562.

Ahmed, M; Bjurholm, A; Theodorsson, E; Schultzberg, M; Kreicbergs, A. Neuropeptide Y- and vasoactive intestinal polypeptide-like immunoreactivity in adjuvant arthritis: effects of capsaicin treatment. *Neuropeptides,* 1995, 29, 33-43.

Ahmed, S; Wang, N; Hafeez, BB; Cheruvu, VK; Haqqi, TM. Punica granatum L. extract inhibits IL-1beta-induced expression of matrix metalloproteinases by inhibiting the activation of MAP kinases and NF-kappaB in human chondrocytes *in vitro*. *J Nutr,* 2005, 135, 2096-2102.

Albright, AL; Gilmartin, R; Swift, P; Krach, LE; Ivanhoe, CB; McLaughlin, JF. Long term intrathecal baclofen therapy for severe spasticity of cerebral origin. *J Neurosurg,* 2003, 98, 291-295.

Aley, KO; Green, PG; Levine, JD. Opioid and adenosine peripheral antinociception are subject to tolerance and withdrawal. *J Neurosci,* 1995, 15, 8031-8038.

Allan, L; Richarz, U; Simpson, K; Slappendel, R. Transdermal fentanyl versus sustained release oral morphine in strong-opioid naïve patients with chronic low back pain. *Spine,* 2005, 30, 2484-2490.

Almekinders, LC; Baynes, AJ; Bracey, LW. An in vitro investigation into the effects of repetitive motion and nonsteroidal antiinflammatory medication on human tendon fibroblasts. *Am J Sports Med,* 1995, 23,119-23.

Al-Nammari, SS; Lucas, JD; Lam, KS. Hematogenous methicillin-resistant Staphylococcus aureus spondylodiscitis. *Spine*, 2007, 32, 2480-2486.

Alvarez, DJ; Rockwell, PG. Trigger points: diagnosis and management. *Am Fam Physician*, 2002, 65, 653-660.

Amara, SG; Jonas, V; Rosenfeld, MG; Ong, ES; Evans, RM. Alternative RNA processing in calcitonin gene expression generates mRNAs encoding different polypeptide products. *Nature*, 1982, 298, 240–244.

American Chiropractic Association. Policy Statement on Spinal Manipulation. February 2003. Available at: http://www.acatoday.com/content_css.cfm?CID=1083.Accessed April 16, 2007.

Ammon, HP; Safayhi, H; Mack, T; Sabieraj, J. Mechanism of antiinflammatory actions of curcumine and boswellic acids. *J Ethnopharmacol,* 1993, 38:113-119.

Andersson, HI; Ejlertsson, G; Leden, I; Rosenberg, C. Chronic pain in a geographically defined general population: studies of differences in age, gender, social class and pain localization. *Clin J Pain*, 1993, 9, 174-182.

Anderson, VC; Burchiel, KJ. A prospective study of long-term intrathecal morphine in the management of chronic nonmalignant pain. *Neurosurgery*, 1999, 44, 289-300.

Anderson, VC; Cooke, B; Burchiel, KJ. Intrathecal hydromorphone for chronic nonmalignant pain: A retrospective study. *Pain Med*, 2001, 2, 287-297.

Arita, M; Bianchini, F; Aliberti, J; Sher, A; Chiang, N; Hong, S; Yang, R; Petasis, NA; Serhan, CN. Stereochemical assignment, antiinflammatory properties, and receptor for the omega-3 lipid mediator resolvin E1. *J Exp Med*, 2005, 201, 713−722.

Arun, R; Kasbekar, AV; Mehdian, SM. Spontaneous kyphotic collapse followed by autostabilisation secondary to cervical osteomyelitis in an intravenous drug abuser. *Acta Orthop Belg*, 2007, 73, 807-811.

Assendelft, WJ; Morton, SC; Yu, EI; Suttorp, MJ; Shekelle, PG. Spinal manipulative therapy for low back pain: a meta-analysis of effectiveness relative to other therapies. *Ann Intern Med*, 2003, 138: 871-881

Astin, JA; Beckner, W; Soeken, K; Hochberg, MC; Berman, B. Psychological interventions for rheumatoid arthritis: a meta-analysis of randomized controlled trials. *Arthritis Rheum*, 2002, 47, 291-302.

Bablis, P; Pollard, H; Bonello, R. Neuro Emotional Technique for the treatment of trigger point sensitivity in chronic neck pain sufferers: A controlled clinical trial. *Chiropractic and Osteopathy*, 2008, 16, 4.

Baker, AS; Ojemann, RG; Swartz, MN; Richardson, EP. Spinal epidural abscess. *N Engl J Med*, 1975, 293, 463-468.

Baker, R; Dreyfuss, P; Mercer, S; Bogduk, N. Cervical transforaminal injection of corticosteroids into a radicular artery: a possible mechanism for spinal cord injury. *Pain*, 2003, 103, 211-215.

Barcelo, HA; Wiemeyer, JC; Sagasta, CL; Macias, M; Barreira, JC. Effect of S-adenosylmethionine on experimental osteoarthritis in rabbits. *Am J Med*, 1987, 83, 55-59.

Barnes, PJ; Belvisi, MG; Rogers, DF. Modulation of neurogenic inflammation: novel approaches to inflammatory disease. *Trends Pharmacol Sci*, 1990, 11,185-189.

Barton, E; Flanagan, P; Hill, S. Spinal infection caused by ESBL-producing Klebsiella pneumoniae treated with Temocillin. *J Infect*, 2008, 57, 347-349.

Baron, JA; Sandler, RS; Bresalier, RS; Lanas, A; Morton, DG; Riddell, R; Iverson, ER; Demets, DL. Cardiovascular events associated with rofecoxib: final analysis of the APPROVe trial. *Lancet*, 2008, 372, 1756-1764.

Barontini, F; Conti, P; Marello, G; Maurri, S. Major neurological sequelae of lumbar epidural anesthesia. Report of three cases. *Ital J Neurol Sci*, 1996, 17, 333-339.

Bassetti, M; Vitale, F; Melica, G; Righi, E; Di Biagio, A; Molfetta, L; Pipino, F; Cruciani, M; Bassetti, D. Linezolid in the treatment of Gram-positive prosthetic joint infections. *J Antimicrob Chemother*, 2005, 55, 387-390.

Bassleer, C Rovati, L; Franchimont, P. Stimulation of proteoglycan production by glucosamine sulfate in chondrocytes isolated from human osteoarthritic articular cartilage in vitro. *Osteoarthritis Cartilage*, 1998, 6, 427-434.

Belfrage, M; Segerdahl, M; Arnér, S; Sollevi, A. The safety and efficacy of intrathecal adenosine in patients with chronic neuropathic pain. *Anesth. Analg*, 1999, 89, 136-142.

Berbari, EF; Steckelberg, JM; Osmon, DR. Osteomyelitis. In: Mandell GL, Bennett JE, Dolin R, eds. *Mandell, Douglas, and Bennett's Principles and Practice of Infectious Diseases.* 6th ed. Oxford, England: Churchill Livingstone.; 2005:1322-1330.

Berg, HE; Berggren, G; Tesch, P. Dynamic neck strength training effect on pain and function. *Archives of Physical Medicine and Rehabilitation*, 1994, 75, 661–665.

Bernard, JM; Macaire, P. Dose-range effects of clonidine added to lidocaine for brachial plexus block. *Anesthesiology*, 1997, 87, 277-284.

Besson, M; Desmeals, J; Piguet, V. What is the place of topical analgesia in neuropathic pain. *Rev Med*, 2008, 4, 1500, 1502-1504.

Bihari, K. Safety, effectiveness, and duration of effect of BOTOX after switching from Dysport for blepharospasm, cervical dystonia, and hemifacial spasm dystonia, and hemifacial spasm. *Curr Med Res Opin*, 2005, 21, 433-438.

Birrell, GJ; McQueen, DS; Iggo, A; Coleman, RA; Grubb, BD. PGI2-induced activation and sensitization of articular mechanonociceptors. *Neurosci Lett*, 1991,124, 5-8.

Black, JA; Liu, S; Tanaka, M; Cummins, TR; Waxman, SG. Changes in the expression of tetrodotoxin-sensitive sodium channels within dorsal root ganglia neurons in inflammatory pain. *Pain*, 2004, 108, 237-247.

Blossfeldt, P. Acupuncture for chronic neck pain--a cohort study in an NHS pain clinic. *Acupunct. Med.*, 2004, 22,146-151.

Bonnefont, J; Alloui, A; Chapuy, E; Clottes, E; Eschalier, A. Orally administered paracetamol does not act locally in the rat formalin test: evidence for a supraspinal, serotonin-dependent antinociceptive mechanism. *Anesthesiology*, 2003, 99, 976-981.

Bonnefont, J; Chapuy, E; Clottes, E; Alloui, A; Eschalier, A. Spinal 5-HT1A receptors differentially influence nociceptive processing according to the nature of the noxious stimulus in rats: effect of WAY-100635 on the antinociceptive activities of paracetamol, venlafaxine and 5-HT. *Pain*, 2005,114, 482-490.

Bonnetfont, J; Daulhac, L; Etienne, M; Chapuy, E; Mallet, C; Ouchuchane,L; Deval, C; Courade, J-P; ferrara, M; Eschalier, A; Clottes, E. Acetaminophen recruits spinal p42/p44 MAPKs and HH/IGF-1 receptors to produce analgesia via the serotonergic system. *Mol Pharmacol*, 2007, 71, 407-415.

Bono, G; Antonaci, F; Ghirmai, S; D'Angelo, F; Berger, M; Nappi, G. Whiplash injuries: clinical picture and diagnostic work-up. *Clin Exp Rheumatol*, 2000, 18(2 Suppl 19), S23-28.

Bot, SD; Terwee, CB; van der Windt, DA; Bouter, LM; Dekker, J; de Vet, HC. Clinimetric evaluation of shoulder disability questionnaires: a systematic review of the literature. *Ann Rheum Dis*, 2004, 63, 335-341.

Bot, SD; van der Waal, JM; Terwee, CB; van der Windt, DA; Schellevis, FG; Bouter, LM; Dekker, J. Incidence and prevalence of complaints of the neck and upper extremity in general practice. *Ann Rheum Dis*, 2005, 64, 118-123.

Borman, P; Keskin, D; Ekici, B; Bodur, H. The efficacy of intermittent cervical traction in patents with chronic neck pain. *Clin Rheumatol*, 2008, 27, 1249-1253.

Börsbo, B; Peolsson, M; Gerdle, B. Catastrophizing, depression, and pain: Correlation with and influence on quality of life and health - A study of chronic whiplash-associated disorders. *J Rehabil Med*, 2008, 40, 562-569.

Braker, C; Yariv, S; Adler, R; Badarny, S; Eisenberg, E. The analgesic effect of botulinum-toxin A on postwhiplash neck pain. *Clin J Pain*, 2008, 24, 5-10.

Braun, J; McHugh, N; Singh, A; Wajdula, JS; Sato, R. Improvement in patient-reported outcomes for patients with ankylosing spondylitis treated with etanercept 50 mg once-weekly and 25 mg twice weekly. *Rheumatology* (Oxford), 2007, 46, 999-1004.

Breit, R; Nade, S .Pseudomonas osteomyelitis of the spine. Report of a case not associated with drug abuse. *Aust N Z J Surg* 1987, 57, 871-873.

Brimijoin, S; Helland, L. Rapid retrograde transport of dopamine-B-hydroxylase as examined by stop-flow technique. *Brain Res*, 1976, 102, 217-228.

Bronfort, G; Evans, R; Nelson, B; Aker, PD; Goldsmith, CH; Vernon, H. A randomized clinical trial of exercise and spinal manipulation for patients with chronic neck pain. *Spine*, 2001, 26, 788–797.

Brook, I. Two cases of diskitis attributable to anaerobic bacteria in children. *Pediatrics*, 2001,107, E26.

Brouwers, PJ; Kottink, EJ; Simon, MA; Prevo, RL. A cervical anterior spinal artery syndrome after diagnostic blockade of the right C6-nerve root. *Pain*, 2001, 91, 397-399.

Brown, AM; Edwards, CM; Davey, MR; Power, JB; Lowe, KC. Pharmacological activity of feverfew (Tanacetum parthenium [L.] Schultz-Bip.): assessment by inhibition of human polymorphonuclear leukocyte chemiluminescence in vitro. *J Pharm Pharmacol*, 1997, 49, 558-561.

Browning, R; Jackson, JL; O'Malley, PG. Cyclobenzaprine and back pain. A Meta analysis. *Arch. Int. Med.*, 2001, 161, 1613-1620.

Bruyere, O; Reginster, JY. Glucosamine and chondroitin sulfate as therapeutic agents for knee and hip osteoarthritis. *Drugs Aging*, 2007, 24, 573-580.

Bush, K; Hillier, S. Outcome of cervical radiculopathy treated with periradicular/epidural corticosteroid injections: a prospective study with independent clinical review. *Eur Spine J*, 1996, 5, 319-325.

Buskila, D; Neumann, L; Vaisberg, G; Alkalay, D; Wolfe, F. Increased rates of fibromyalgia following cervical spine injury. A controlled study of 161 cases of traumatic injury. *Arthritis Rheum*, 1997, 40, 446-452.

Bustamante, D; Paeile, C; Willer, JC; Le Bars, D. Effects of intravenous nonsteroidal antiinflammatory drugs on a C-fiber reflex elicited by a wide range of stimulus intensities in the rat. *J Pharmacol Exp Ther*, 1996, 276, 1232-1243.

Cano, SJ; Hobart, JC; Edwards, M; Fitzpatrick, R; Bhatia, K; Thompson, AJ; Warner, TT. CDIP-58 can measure the impact of botulinum toxin treatment in cervical dystonia. *Neurology*, 2006, 67, 2230-2232.

Capasso, F; Balestrieri, B; Di Rosa, M; Persico, P; Sorrentino, L. Enhancement of carrageenin foot oedema by 1,10 -phenanthroline and evidence for the bradykinin as endogenous mediator. *Agents Actions*, 1975, 5, 359-363.

Carlsson, KC; Hoem, NO; Moberg, ER; Mathisen, LC. Analgesic effect of dextromethorphan in neuropathic pain. *Acta Anaesthesiol Scand*, 2004, 48, 328-336.

Carron H. Relieving pain with nerve blocks. *Geriatrics* 1978, 33, 49-57.

Carter, MS; Krause, JE. Structure, expression, and some regulatory mechanisms of the rat preprotachykinin gene encoding substance P, neurokinin A, neuropeptide K, and neuropeptide gamma. *J Neurosci*, 1990, 10, 2203–2214.

Caterina, MJ; Schumacher, MA; Tominaga, M; Rosen, TA; Levine, JD; Julius D. The capsaicin receptor: a heat-activated ion channel in the pain pathway. *Nature*, 1997, 389(6653), 816-824.

Caterina, MJ; Leffler, A; Malmberg, AB; Martin, WJ; Trafton, J; Petersen-Zeitz, KR; Koltzenburg, M; Basbaum, AI; Julius, D. Impaired nociception and pain sensation in mice lacking the capsaicin receptor. *Science*, 2000, 288, 306–313.

Cazalets, JR; Bertrand, S; squalli-Houssaini, Y; Clarac, F. GABAergic control of spinal locomotor networks in the neonatal rat. *Ann. N Y Acad Sci*, 1998, 860, 168-180.

Chan, PS; Caron, JP; Orth, MW. Short-term gene expression changes in cartilage explants stimulated with interleukin beta plus glucosamine and chondroitin sulfate. *J Rheumatol*, 2006, 33, 1329-1340.

Chan, PS; Caron, JP; Orth, MW. Effect of glucosamine and chondroitin sulfate on regulation of gene expression of proteolytic enzymes and their inhibitors in interleukin-1-challenged bovine articular cartilage explants. *Am J Vet Res*, 2005, 66, 1870-1876.

Chandrasekharan, NV; Dai, H; Roos, KL; Evanson, NK; Tomsik, J; Elton, TS; Simmons, DL. COX-3, a cyclooxygenase-1 variant inhibited by acetaminophen and other analgesic/ antipyretic drugs: cloning, structure, and expression. *Proc Natl Acad Sci USA*, 2002, 99, 13926-13931.

Chao J. Retrospective analysis of Kadian (morphine sulfate sustained-release capsules) in patients with chronic, nonmalignant pain. *Pain Med,* 2005, 6, 262-265.

Chiang, N; Arita, M; Serhan, CN. Anti-inflammatory circuitry: lipoxin, aspirin-triggered lipoxins and their receptor ALX. *Prostaglandins Leukot Essent Fatty Acids*, 2005, 73(3-4), 163-177.

Childers, MK; Borenstein, D; Brown, RL; Gershon, S; Hale, ME; Petri, M; Wan, GJ; Laudadio, C; Harrison, DD. Low-dose cyclobenzaprine versus combination therapy with ibuprofen for acute neck or back pain with muscle spasm: a randomized trial. *Curr Med Res Opin*, 2005, 21,1485-1493.

Chou, R; Qaseem, A; Snow, V; Casey, D; Cross, JT; Shekelle, P; Owens, DK. Diagnosis and treatment of low back pain: a joint clinical practice guideline from the American College of Physicians and the American Pain Society. *Ann. Intern Med*, 2007, 147, 478-491.

Cibere, J; Kopec, JA; Thorne, A; Singer, J; Canvin, J; Robinson, DB; Pope, J; Hong, P; Grant, E; Esdaile, JM. Randomized, double-blind, placebo-controlled glucosamine discontinuation trial in knee osteoarthritis. *Arthritis Rheum*, 2004, 51, 738-745.

Civelli, O; Nothacker, HP; Reinscheid, R. Reverse physiology: discovery of the novel neuropeptide, orphanin FQ/nociceptin. *Crit Rev Neurobiol*, 1998, 12, 163-176.

Classen, AM; Wimbish, GH; Kupiec, TC. Stability of admixture containing morphine sulfate, bupivacaine hydrochloride, and clonidine hydrochloride in an implantable infusion system. *J Pain Symptom Manage*, 2004, 28,603-611.

Cluzel, RA; Lopitaux, R; Sirot, J; Rampon, S. Rifampicin in the treatment of osteoarticular infections due to staphylococci. *J Antimicrob Chemother*, 1984, 13(suppl c), 23-29.

Cohen, RH; Perl, ER. Contributions of arachidonic acid derivatives and substance P to the sensitization of cutaneous nociceptors. *J Neurophysiol*, 1990, 64, 457-464.

Cohen, SP; Chang, AS; Larkin, T; Mao, J. The intravenous ketamine test: A predictive response tool for oral dextromethorphan treatment in neuropathic pain. *Anesth Analg*, 2004, 99, 1753-1759.

Cohen, SP; Wang, S; Chen, L; Kurihara, C; McKnight, G; Marcuson, M; Mao, J. An Intravenous Ketamine Test as a Predictive Response Tool in Opioid-Exposed Patients with Persistent Pain. *J Pain Symptom Manage*, 2008 Sep 11

Colbert, AP; Wahbeh, H; Harling, N; Connelly, E; Schiffke, HC; Forsten, C; Gregory, WL; Markov, MS; Souder, JJ; Elmer, P; King, V. Static magnetic field therapy: A critical review of treatment parameters. *Evid Based Complement Alternat Med* 2007 Oct 4.

Collier, HO; Butt, NM; McDonald-Gibson, WJ; Saeed, SA. Extract of feverfew inhibits prostaglandin biosynthesis. *Lancet*, 1980, 2, 922-923.

Conaughty, JM; Chen, J; Martinez, OV; Chiappetta, G; Brookfield, KF; Eismont, F. Efficacy of linezolid versus vancomycin in the treatment of methicillin-resistant staphylococcus aureus discitis: a controlled animal model. *Spine*, 2006, 31, E830-E832.

Corning, JL. Spinal anesthesia and local medication of the cord. *N Y Med J*, 1885, 42, 483-485.

Costa, J; Espírito-Santo, C; Borges, A; Ferreira, JJ; Coelho, M; Moore, P; Sampaio, C. Botulinum toxin type B for cervical dystonia. *Cochrane Database of Systematic Reviews*, 2004, Issue 4. Art. No.: CD004315. DOI: 10.1002/14651858.CD004315.pub2.

Côté, P; Cassidy, JD; Carroll, L: The Saskatchewan Health and Back Pain Survey: The prevalence of neck pain and related disability in Saskatchewan adults. *Spine*, 1998, 23, 1689-1698.

Côté, P; Cassidy, JD; Carroll, L. The factors associated with neck pain and its related disability in the Saskatchewan population. *Spine*, 2000, 25, 1109-1117.

Côté, P; Cassidy, JD; Carroll L. The treatment of neck and low back pain: who seeks care? who goes where? *Med Care*, 2001, 39, 956-967.

Cottle, L; Riordan, T. Infectious spondylodiscitis. *J Infect*, 2008, 56, 401-412.

Courade, JP; Chassaing, C; Bardin, L; Alloui, A; Eschalier, A. 5-HT receptor subtypes involved in the spinal antinociceptive effect of acetaminophen in rats. *Eur J Pharmacol*, 2001, 432, 1-7.

Cousins, DV; Wilton, SD; Francis, BR; Gow, BL. Use of polymerase chain reaction for rapid diagnosis of tuberculosis. *J Clin Microbiol*, 1992, 30, 255-258.

Crawley, B; Saito, O; Malkmus, S; Fitzsimmons, B; Hua, X-Y; Yaksh, TL. Acetaminophen prevents hyperalgesia in central pain cascade. *Neurosci Lett*, 2008, 442, 50-53.

Crowley, KL. Clinical application of ketamine ointment in the treatment of sympathetically maintained pain. *Int J Pharm Compound*, 1998, 2, 122–127.

Currier BL: Spinal infections. In: An HS (ed). *Principles and Techniques of Spine Surgery*. Baltimore: Williams and Wilkins; 1998; 567-603.

Dagenais, S; Yelland, MJ; Del Mar, C; Schoene, ML Prolotherapy injections for chronic low-back pain. *Cochrane Database Syst Rev*, 2007, (2), CD004059.

Dahl, JB; Kehlet, H. Non-steroidal anti-inflammatory drugs: rationale for use in severe postoperative pain. *Br J Anaesth,* 1991, 66, 703-712.

Danner, RL; Hartman, BJ. Update on spinal epidural abscess: 35 cases and review of the literature. *Rev Infect Dis*, 1987, 9, 265-274.

Darland, T; Heinriche,r MM; Grandy, DK. Orphanin FQ/nociceptin: a role in pain and analgesia, but so much more. *Trends Neurosci*, 1998, 21, 215-221.

Darlington, LG; Stone, TW. Antioxidants and fatty acids in the amelioration of rheumatoid arthritis and related disorders. *Br J Nutr*, 2001, 85, 251-269.

De Kock, M; Gautier, P; Pavlopoulou, A; Jonniaux, M; Lavand'homme, P. Epidural clonidine or bupivacaine as the sole analgesic agent during and after abdominal surgery: a comparative study. *Anesthesiology*, 1999, 90, 1354-1362. Erratum in: *Anesthesiology*, 1999, 91, 602.

De Felipe, C; Herrero, JF; O'Brien, JA; Palmer, JA; Doyle, CA; Smith, AJ; Laird, JM; Belmonte, C; Cervero, F; Hunt, SP. Altered nociception, analgesia and aggression in mice lacking the receptor for substance P. *Nature*, 1998, 392, 394-397.

de Goeij, S; Nisolle, JF; Glupczynski, Y; Delgrange, E; Delaere, B. Vertebral osteomyelitis with spinal epidural abscess in two patients with Bacteroides fragilis bacteraemia. *Acta Clin Belg*, 2008, 63, 193-196.

de Las Peñas, CF; Alonso-Blanco, C; Miangolarra, JC. Myofascial trigger points in subjects presenting with mechanical neck pain: A blinded, controlled study. *Man Ther*, 2007, 12, 29-33.

de Las Peñas, CF; Alonso-Blanco, C; Cleland, JA; Rodríguez-Blanco, C; Alburquerque-Sendín, F. Changes in pressure pain thresholds over C5-C6 zygapophyseal joint after a cervicothoracic junction manipulation in healthy subjects. *J Manipulative Physiol Ther*, 2008, 31, 332-337.

Dellemijn, PL; Vanneste, JA. Randomised double-blind active-placebo-controlled crossover trial of intravenous fentanyl in neuropathic pain. *Lancet*, 1997, 349(9054), 753-758.

Denti, M; Randelli, P; Bigoni, M; Vitale, G; Marino, MR; Fraschini, N. Pre- and postoperative intra-articular analgesia for arthroscopic surgery of the knee and arthroscopy-assisted anterior cruciate ligament reconstruction. A double-blind randomized, prospective study. *Knee Surg Sports Traumatol Arthrosc*, 1997, 5, 206-212.

Deutsch, DG; Chin, SA. Enzymatic synthesis and degradation of anandamide, a cannabinoid receptor agonist. *Biochem Pharmacol*, 1993, 46, 791-796.

Dickenson AH. Enkephalins. A new approach to pain relief? *Nature*, 1986, 320(6064), 681-682.

Dickenson, AH. Spinal cord pharmacology of pain. *Br J Anaesth*, 1995, 75, 193-200.

Dickenson, AH; Sullivan, AF; Stanfa, LC; McQuay, HJ. Dextromethorphan and levorphanol on dorsal horn nociceptive neurons in the rat. *Neuropharmacology*, 1991, 30, 1303–1308.

Dimar, JR; Carreon, LY; Glassman, SD; Campbell, MJ; Hartman, MJ; Johnson, JR. Treatment of pyogenic vertebral osteomyelitis with anterior debridement and fusion followed by delayed posterior spinal fusion. *Spine*, 2004, 29, 326-332.

DiMarzo, V; Bisogno, T; DePetrocellis, L. Anandamide: some like it hot. *Trends Pharmacol Sci.*, 2001, 22, 346-349.

Dodge, GR Jimenez, SA. Glucosamine sulfate modulates the levels of aggrecan and matrix metalloproteinase-3 synthesized by cultured human osteoarthritis articular chondrocytes. *Osteoarthritis Cart*, 2003, 11, 424-432.

Donnerer, J; Schuligoi, R; Stein, C. Increased content and transport of substance P and calcitonin gene-related peptide in sensory nerves innervating inflamed tissue: evidence for a regulatory function of nerve growth factor in vivo. *Neuroscience*, 1992, 49, 693–698.

Dornan, WA; Vink, KL; Malen, P; Short, K; Struthers, W; Barrett, C. Site-specific effects of intracerebral injections of three neurokinins (neurokinin A, neurokinin K, and neurokinin gamma) on the expression of male rat sexual behavior. *Physiol Behav*, 1993, 54, 249–258.

Dray, A. Inflammatory mediators of pain. *Br. J. Anaesth*, 1995, 75, 125-131.

Dray, A. Kinins and their receptors in hyperalgesia. *Can J Pharmacol*, 1997, 75, 704-712.

Dray, A; Rang, H. The how and why of chronic pain states and the what of new analgesia therapies. *Trends Neurosci*, 1998, 2, 315-317.

Dressler, D; Hallett, M. Immunological aspects of Botox, Dyport and Mybloc/Neurobloc. *Eur J Neurol*, 2006, 13 suppl 1, 11-15.

Dualé, C; Daveau, J; Cardot, JM; Boyer-Grand, A; Schoeffler,P; Dubray, C. Cutaneous amitriptyline in human volunteers: differential effects on the components of sensory information. *Anesthesiology*, 2008,108, 714-721.

Duggan, AW; Hope, PJ; Jarrott, B; Schaible, HG; Fleet-Wood,SM. Release, spread and persistenceof immunoreactive neurokininA in the dorsal hornof the cat following noxious cutaneous stimulation. Studies with antibody microprobes. *Neuroscience*, 1990, 35, 195-202.

Dykstra, DD; Mendez, A; Chaauis, D; Baxter, T; Deslauriers, L; Stuckey, M. Treatment of cervical dystonia and focal hand dystonia by high cervical continuously infused intrathecal baclofen; a report of 2 cases. *Arch Phys Med Rehabil*, 2005, 86, 830-833.

Eaton, M J; Karmally, S; Martinez, MA; Plunkett, JA; Lopez, T; Cejas, PJ. *J Periphery Nerv Syst*, 1999, 4, 245–257.

Edvinsson, L. New therapeutic target in primary headaches – blocking the CGRP receptor. *Expert Opin Ther Targets*, 2003, 7, 377–383.

Eisenach, JC. Muscarinic-mediated analgesia. *Life Sci*, 1999, 64, 549-554.

Eismont, FJ; Bohlman, HH; Soni, PL; Goldberg, VM; Freehafer AA. Pyogenic and fungal vertebral osteomyelitis with paralysis. *J Bone Joint Surg Am*, 1983, 65,19-29.

Ellrich, J; Makowska, A. Nerve growth factor and ATP excite different neck muscle nociceptors in anaesthetized mice. *Cephalalgia*, 2007, 27, 1226-1235.

Endress, C; Guyot, DR; Fata, J; Salciccioli, G. Cervical osteomyelitis due to i.v. heroin use: radiologic findings in 14 patients. *Am J Roentgenol*, 1990, 155, 333-335.

England, S; Bevan, S; Docherty, RJ. PGE2 modulates the tetrodotoxin-resistant sodium current in neonatal rat dorsal root ganglion neurones via the cyclic AMP-protein kinase A cascade. *J Physiol*, 1996, 495(Pt 2), 429-40.

Ernst, E; Chrubasik, S. Phyto-anti-inflammatories: a systematic review of randomized, placebo-controlled, double blind trials. *Rheum Dis Clin North Am*, 2000, 1, 13-27.

Ernst, E. The efficacy of Phytodolor for the treatment of musculoskeletal pain -- a systematic review of randomized clinical trials. *Nat Med J*, 1999, 2, 14-17.

Ernst, E. Usage of complementary therapies in rheumatology. A systematic review. *Clin Rheumatol*, 1998, 17, 301-305.

Ernst, E; Pittler, MH; Stevinson, C; White, AR. *The Desktop Guide to Complementary and Alternative Medicine*. Edinburgh: Mosby; 2001.

Ernst, E. Avacodo-soybean unsaponifiables (ASU) for osteoarthritis -- a systematic review. *Clin Rheumatol*, 2003, 22, 285-288.

Fass, RJ. Treatment of osteomyelitis and septic arthritis with cefazolin. *Antimicrob Agents Chemother*, 1978, 13, 405-411.

Fejer, R; Kyvik, KO; Hartvigsen, J: The prevalence of neck pain in the world population: a systematic critical review of the literature. *Eur Spine J*, 2006, 15, 834-848.

Ferrante, FM; Bearn, L; Rothrock, R; King, L. Evidence against trigger point injection technique for the treatment of cervicothoracic myofacial pain with with botulinium toxin type A. *Anesthsiology*, 2005, 103, 377-383.

Fischer, AA. Pressure threshold meter: its use for quantification of tender spots. *Arch Phys Med Rehabil*, 1986, 67, 836-838.

Fitzgerald, M; Woolf, CJ. The time course and specificity of the changes in the behavioural and dorsal horn cell responses to noxious stimuli following peripheral nerve capsaicin treatment in the rat. *Neuroscience*, 1982, 7, 2051–2056.

Forestier, R; Françon, A; Saint, Arroman, F; Bertolino, C. French version of the Copenhagen neck functional disability scale. *Joint Bone Spine*, 2007, 74, 155-159.

França, DL; Senna-Fernandes, V; Cortez, CM; Jackson, MN; Bernardo-Filho, M; Guimarães, MA. Tension neck syndrome treated by acupuncture combined with physiotherapy: A comparative clinical trial (pilot study). *Complement Ther Med*, 2008, 16, 268-277.

Frank, C; Amiel, D; Woo, SL-Y; Akeson, W. Normal ligament properties and ligament healing. *Clin Ortho Res* 1985, 196, 15-25.

Freund, BJ; Schwartz, M. Treatment of whiplash associated neck pain [corrected] with botulinum toxin-A: a pilot study. *J Rheumatol*, 2000, 27, 481-484.

Frondoza, CG; Sohrabi, A; Polotsky, A; Phan, PV; Hungerford, DS; Lindmark, L. An in vitro screening assay for inhibitors of proinflammatory mediators in herbal extracts using human synoviocyte cultures. *In Vitro Cell Dev Biol Anim*, 2004, 40, 95-101.

Fuentes, JA; Ruiz-Gayo, M; Manzanares, J; Vela, G; Reche, I; Corchero, J. Cannabinoids as potential new analgesics. *Life Sci*, 1999, 65, 675-685.

Ga, H; Choi, JH; Park, CH; Yoon, HJ. Acupuncture needling versus lidocaine injection of trigger points in myofascial pain syndrome in elderly patients--a randomised trial. *Acupunct Med*, 2007, 25, 130-136.

Gagnier, JJ; Van Tulder, MW; Berman, B; Bombardier, C. Herbal medicine for low back pain: a Cochrane review. *Spine*, 2007, 32, 82-92.

Gaillard JM. Comparison of two muscle relaxant drugs on human sleep: diazepam and parachlorophenylgaba. *Acta Psychiatr Belg*, 1977, 77, 410-425.

Gaumann, DM; Brunet, BC; Jirounek, P. Hyperpolarization after potentials in C-fibers and local anesthetic effects of clonidine and lidocaine. *Pharmacology*, 1994, 48, 21-29.

Gaumann, D; Forster, A; Griessen, M; Habre, W; Poinsot, O; Della Santa, D. Comparison between clonidine and epinephrine admixture to lidocaine in brachial plexus block. *Anesth Analg*, 1992, 75, 69-74.

Gazerani, P; Staahl, C; Drewes, AM; Arendt-Nielsen, L. The effects of Botulinum Toxin type A on capsaicin-evoked pain, flare, and secondary hyperalgesia in an experimental human model of trigeminal sensitization. *Pain*, 2006, 122, 315-325.

Genevay, S; Stingelin, S. Efficacy of etanercept in the treatment of acute, severe sciatica : a pilot study. *Annals of the Rheumatic Diseases*, 2004, 63, 1120-1123.

Gerwin, RD. Myofascial and visceral pain syndromes: visceral somatic pain representations. *J Musculoskeletal Pain*, 2002, 10, 165-175.

Gilron, I; Booher, SL; Rowan, MS; Smoller, MS; Max, MB. A randomized, controlled trial of high-dose dextromethorphan in facial neuralgias. *Neurology*, 2000, 55, 964-971.

Gorchakova, TV; Suprun, IV; Sobenin, IA; Orekhov, AN. Use of natural products in anticytokine therapy. *Bull Exp Biol Med*, 2007, 143, 316-319.

Gottrup, H; Bach, FW; Arendt-Nielsen, L; Jensen, TS. Peripheral lidocaine but not ketamine inhibits capsaicin-induced hyperalgesia in humans. *Br J Anaesth*, 2000, 85, 520-528.

Gottrup, H; Bach, FW; Jensen, TS. Differential effects of peripheral ketamine and lidocaine on skin flux and hyperalgesia induced by intradermal capsaicin in humans. *Clin. Physiol Funct Imaging*, 2004, 24, 103-108.

Graziani, AL; Lawson, LA; Gibson, GA; Steinberg, MA; MacGregor, RR. Vancomycin concentrations in infected and noninfected human bone. *Antimicrob Agents Chemother*, 1988, 32, 1320-1322.

Guo, YQ; Chen, LY; Fu, WB; Xu, MZ; Ou, XM. Clinically randomized controlled study on abdominal acupuncture for treatment of cervical spondylosis. *Zhongguo Zhen Jiu*, 2007, 27, 652-656.

Gureje, O; Akinpelu, AO; Uwakwe, R; Udofia, O; Wakil, A. Comorbidity and impact of chronic spinal pain in Nigeria. *Spine*, 2007, 32, E495-500.

Gutierrez, S; Palacios, I; Sanchez-Pernaute, O; Hernández, P; Moreno, J; Egido, J; Herrero-Beaumont, G. SAMe restores the changes in the proliferation and in the synthesis of fibronectin and proteoglycans induced by tumour necrosis factor alpha on cultured rabbit synovial cells. *Br J Rheumatol*, 1997, 36, 27-31.

Guyader, M. Les palantes antirheumatismales. Etudes historique et pharmalogique, et etude clinique du nebulisat d'Harpagophytum procumbens DC chez 50 patients arthroques sulvis en service hospitalier. Paris: Universite Pierre et Marie Curie; 1984. (Dissertation).

Hackett G. Low back pain. *Indust Med Surg*, 1959, 28, 416-419.

Hackett, G; Hemwall, G; Montgomery, G. *Ligament and tendon relaxation treated by prolotherapy*. 5th ed. Gustav A. Hemwall; Oak Park, IL; 1992.

Hadjipavlou, AG; Mader, JT; Necessary, JT; Muffoletto, AJ. Hematogenous pyogenic spinal infections and their surgical management. *Spine*, 2000, 25, 1668-1679.

Haines, T; Gross, A; Goldsmith, CH; Perry, L. Patient education for neck pain with or without radiculopathy. *Cochrane Database Syst Rev*, 2008, (4):CD005106.

Hansen, C; Gilron, I; Hong, M. The effect of intrathecal gabapentinon spinal morphine tolerance in rat tail-flickand paw pressure test. *Anesth analg*, 2004, 99,1180-1184.

Hansson, E; Hansson, T; Jonsson, R. Predictors for work ability and disability in men and women with low-back or neck problems. *Eur Spine J*, 2006, 15, 780-793.

Hanten, WP; Olsen, SL; Butts, NL; Nowicki, AL. Effectiveness of a home program of ischaemic pressure followed by sustained stretch for treatment of myofascial trigger points. *Phys Ther*, 2000, 80, 997-1003.

Harmand, MF; Vilamitjana, J; Maloche, E; Duphil, R; Ducassou, D: Effects of S-adenosylmethionine on human articular chondrocyte differentiation. An *in vitro* study. *Am J Med*, 1987, 83, 48-54.

Hashimoto, A; Hayashi, I; Murakami, Y; Sato, Y; Kitasato, H; Matsushita, R; Iizuka, N; Urabe, K; Itoman, M; Hirohata, S; Endo, H. Antiinflammatory mediator lipoxin A4 and its receptor in synovitis of patients with rheumatoid arthritis. *J Rheumatol*, 2007, 34, 2144-2153.

Hassenbusch, SJ; Stanton-Hicks, M; Covington, EC; Walsh, JG; Guthrey, DS. Long term intraspinal infusions of opioids in the treatment of neuropathic pain. *J Pain Symptom Manage*, 1995, 10, 527- 543.

Hauser, RA. Punishing the pain. Treating chronic pain with prolotherapy. *Rehab Manag* 1999, 12, 26-28, 30.

Hauser, RA; Hauser, MA. Dextrose prolotherapy for unresolved neck pain. *Practical Pain Management*, 2007, Oct, 56-69.

Hee, HTIII; Whitecloud, TS; Myers, L; Roesch, W; Ricciardi, JE. Do worker's compensation patients with neck pain have lower SF-36 scores? *Eur Spine J*, 2002, 11, 375-381.

Heppelmann B, Pawlak M. Sensitisation of articular afferents in normal and inflamed knee joints by substance P in the rat. *Neurosci Lett*, 1997, 223, 97-100.

Heyneman ,CA; Lawless-Liday, C; Wall, GC. Oral versus topical NSAIDs in rheumatic diseases: a comparison. *Drugs* 2000, 60, 555-574.

Hildebrand, KR; Elsberry, DD; Deer, TR. Stability, compatibility, and safety of intrathecal bupivacaine administered chronically via an implantable delivery system. *Clin J Pain*, 2001, 17, 239-244.

Hinman, M: The therapeutic use of magnets: a review of recent research. *Phys Ther Rev.* 2002, 7, 33-43.

Hirota, K; Lambert, DG. Ketamine: its mechanism(s) of action and unusual clinical uses. *Br J Anaesth*, 1996, 77, 441–444.

Ho, KY; Huh, BK; White, WD; Yeh, CC; Miller, EJ. .Topical amitriptyline versus lidocaine in the treatment of neuropathic pain. *Clin J Pain*, 2008, 24, 51-55.

Hodges, SD; Castleberg, RL; Miller, T; Ward, R; Thorburg, C. Cervical epidural steroid injection with intrinsic spinal cord damage: two case reports. *Spine*, 1998, 23, 2137-2142.

Hogan, KA; Manning, EL; Glaser, JA. Progressive cervical kyphosis associated with botulinum toxin injection. *South Med J*, 2006, 99, 888-891.

Hökfelt, T; Wiesenfeld-Hallin, Z; Villar, M; Melander, T. Increase of galanin-like immunoreactivity in rat dorsal root ganglion cells after peripheral axotomy. *Neurosci. Lett*, 1987, 83, 217-220.

Hökfelt, T; Zhang, X; Wiesenfeld-Hallin, Z. Messenger plasticity in primary sensory neurons following axotomy and its functional implications. *Trends Neurosci*, 1994, 17, 22-30.

Holthusen, H; Arndt, JO. Nitric oxide evokes pain in humans on intracutaneous injection. *Neurosci Lett*, 1994, 165(1-2), 71-74.

Hong, C-Z; Chen, Y-C; Pon, CH; Yu J. Immediate effects of various physical medicine modalities on pain threshold of the active myofascial trigger points. *J Musculoskel Pain*, 1993, 1, 37-52.

Hooper, RA; Frizzell, JB; Faris, P. Case series on chronic whiplash related neck pain treated with intraarticular zygapophysial joint regeneration injection therapy. *Pain Physician*, 2007, 10, 313-318.

Hughes, R; Carr, A. A randomized, double-blind, placebo-controlled trial of glucosamine sulphate as an analgesic in osteoarthritis of the knee. *Rheumatology* (Oxford), 2002, 41, 279-284.

Hsieh, C-YJ; Hong, C-Z. Effect of chiropractic manipulation on the pain threshold of myofascial trigger point. *Proceedings of the 1990 International Conference of Spinal Manipulation: Los Angeles College of Chiropractic; Los Angeles* 1990.

Hsueh, TC; Cheng, PT; Kuan, TS; Hong, CZ. The immediate effectiveness of electrical nerve stimulation and electrical muscle stimulation on myofascial trigger points. *Am J Phys Med Rehabil*, 1997, 76, 471- 476.

Hylden, JKL; Wilcox, GL. Intrathecal substance P elicits a caudally-directed biting and scrathing behavior in mice. *Brain Res*, 1981, 217, 212-215.

Inan, N; Yilmaz, G; Surer, H; Coskun, O; Ucler, S; Cavdar, L; Inan, LE. Is there a role for nitric oxide activity in cervicogenic headache? *Funct Neurol*, 2007, 22, 155-157.

Incavo, SJ; Ronchetti, PJ; Choi, JH; Wu, H; Kinzig, M; Sörgel, F. Penetration of piperacillin-tazobactam into cancellous and cortical bone tissues. *Antimicrob Agents Chemother*, 1994, 38, 905-907.

Inoue, Y; Koga, K; Sata, T; Shigematusa, A. Effect of fentanyl on emergence characteristics from anesthesia in adult cervical spine surgery: a comparison of fentanyl-based and sevoflurane-based anesthesia. *J Anesth*, 2005, 19, 12-16.

Itoh, K; Katsumi, Y; Hirota, S; Kitakoji, H. Randomised trial of trigger point acupuncture compared with other acupuncture for treatment of chronic neck pain. *Complement Ther Med*, 2007, 15, 172-179.

Iversen, L. Substance P equals pain substance? *Nature* 1998, 392, 334-335.

Iversen, LL. Substance P. *Brit Med Bull*, 1982, 38, 277-282.

Iversen, LL; Chapman, V. Cannabinoids: a real prospect for pain relief? *Current Opin Pharmacol*, 2002, 2, 50-55.

Jacobson, S; Danneskield-Samsone, B; Anderson, RB. Oral S-adenosyl methionine in primary fibromyalgia, double-blind clinical evaluation. *Scand J Rheumatol*, 1991, 20, 294-302.

Janda, V. Muscles and motor control in cervicogenic disorders: assessment and management. In: Grant R, editor. *Physical therapy ofthe cervical and thoracic spine*. New York: Churchill Livingstone; 1994;195–216.

Jeal,W; Benfield, P. Transdermal fentanyl. A review of its pharmacological properties and therapeutic efficacy in pain control. *Drugs*, 1997, 53,109-138.

Jensen, AG; Espersen, F; Skinhøj, P; Rosdahl, VT; Frimodt-Møller, N. Increasing frequency of vertebral osteomyelitis following Staphylococcus aureus bacteraemia in Denmark 1980-1990. *J Infect*, 1997, 34,113-118.

Jessell, TM; Iversen, LL. Opiate analgesics inhibit substance P release from rat trigeminal nucleus. *Nature*, 1977, 268(5620), 549-551.

Jhaveri, MD; Elmes, SJ; Richardson, D; Barrett, DA; Kendall, DA; Mason, R; Chapman, V. Evidence for a novel functional role of cannabinoid CB receptors in the thalamus of neuropathic rats. *Eur J Neurosci*, 2008, 27, 1722-1730.

John Hurlebert R. Methylprednisolone for acute spinal cord injury: an inappropriate standard of care. *J Neurosurg (Spine* 1), 2000, 93, 1-7.

Jordan, A; Bendix, T; Nielsen, H; Hansen, F; Host, D; Winkel, A. Intensive training, physiotherapy, or manipulation for patients with chronic neck pain. *Spine*, 1998, 23, 311–319.

Jordan, KM; Arden, NK. EULAR Recommendations 2003: an evidence based approach to the management of knee osteoarthritis: Report of a Task Force of the Standing Committee for International Clinical Studies Including Therapeutic Trials (ESCISIT). *Ann Rheum Dis*, 2003, 62, 1145–1155.

Jull, G; Falla, D; Treleaven, J; Sterling, M;O'Leary, S. A therapeutic exercise approach for cervical disorders. In: *Grieve's modern manual therapy: the vertebral column*, 2004.

Kabat-Zinn, J; Lipworth, I; Burney, R. Four- year follow-up of a meditation-based program for the self regulation of chronic pain: treatment outcomes and compliance. *Clin J Pain*, 1987, 2, 159-173.

Kabat-Zinn, J; Lipworth, I; Burney, R. The clinical use of mindfulness meditation for the self-regulation of chronic pain. *J Behav Med*, 1985, 8, 163-190.

Kang, JD; Georgescu, HI; McIntyre-Larkin, L; Stefanovic-Racic, M; Evans, CH. Herniated cervical intervertebral discs spontaneously produce matrix metalloproteinases, nitric oxide, interleukin-6, and prostaglandin E2. *Spine*, 1995, 20, 2373-2378.

Kangrga, I; Randić, M. Outflow of endogenous aspartate and glutamate from the rat spinal dorsal horn in vitro by activation of low- and high-threshold primary afferent fibers. Modulation by mu-opioids. *Brain Res*, 1991, 553, 347-352.

Kaur, R; Singh, D; Chopra, K. Participation of alpha2 receptors in the antinociceptive activity of quercetin. *J Med Food*, 2005, 8, 529-532.

Kim, K-H; Choi, S-H; Kim, T-K; Shin, SW. Cervical Facet Joint Injections in the Neck and Shoulder Pain. *J. Korean Med Sci*, 2005, 20, 659-662.

Kim, LS; Axelrod, LJ; Howard, P; Buratovich, N; Waters, RF. Efficacy of methylsulfonylmethane (MSM) in osteoarthritis pain of the knee: a pilot clinical trial. *Osteoarthritis Cartilage*, 2006, 14, 286–294.

Kim, SM; Kim, J; Kim, E; Hwang, SJ; Shin, HK; Lee, SE. Local application of capsaicin alleviates mechanical hyperalgesia after spinal nerve transection. *Neurosci Lett*, 2008, 433, 199-204.

Kissin, I; Bright,CA; Bradley, EL. Selective and Long-Lasting Neural Blockade with Resiniferatoxin Prevents Inflammatory Pain Hypersensitivity. *Anesth Analg*, 2002, 94, 1253-1258.

Kissin, I. Vanilloid-induced conduction analgesia: selective, dose dependent, long lasting, with a low level of potential neurotoxicity. *Anesth Analg* 2008,107, 271-281.

Kitahata, LM. Pain pathways and transmission. *Yale J Biol Med* 1993, 66, 437-442.

Klein, G; Kullich, W. Reducing pain by oral enzyme therapy in rheumatic diseases. *Wien Med Wochenschr*, 1999, 149, 577-580.

Klein AW. Complications and adverse reactions with the use of botulinum toxin. *Dis Mon*, 2002, 48, 336-356.

Kohane, DS; Kuang, Y; Lu, NT; Langer, R; Strichartz, GR; Berde CB. Vanilloid receptor agonists potentiate the *in vivo* local anesthetic activity of percutaneously injected site 1 sodium channel blockers. *Anesthesiology*, 1999; 90: 524–34.

Kohlmann T. Epidemiology of orofacial pain. *Schmerz*, 2002, 16, 339-345.

Kolesnikov, Y; Pasternak, GW. Topical opioids in mice: analgesia and reversal of tolerance by a topical N-methyl-D-aspartate antagonist. *J Pharmacol Exp Ther*, 1999, 290, 247-252.

Kolstad, F; Leivseth, G; Nygaard, O. Transforaminal steroid injections in the treatment of cervical radiculopathy. A prospective outcome study. *Acta Neurochi (Wein)*, 2005, 147, 1065-1070.

Kosuge, S; Inagaki, Y; Okumura, H. Studies on the pungent principles of red pepper. Part VIII on the chemical contributions of the pungent principles. *Nippon Nogei Kagaka (J Agri Chem. Soc)* 1961, 35, 923-927.

Kosuge, S; Inagaki, Y. Studies on the pungent principles of red pepper. Part XI. Determination and contents of the two pungent principles. Nippon Nogei Kagaka (*J. Agri. Chem. Soc.*) 1962, 36, 251.

Kovacs, FM; Bago, J; Royuela, A; Seco, J; Gimenez, S. Research Network SB Psychometric characteristics of the Spanish version of instruments to measure neck pain disability. *BMC Musculoskelet Disord*, 2008, 9, 42.

Krames, ES. Intrathecal infusional therapies for intractable pain: Patient management guidelines. *J Pain Symptom Manage*, 1993, 8, 36-46.

Kuraishi, Y; Kawamura, M; Yamaguchi, T; Houtani, T; Kawabata, S; Futaki, S; Fujii, N; Satoh, M. Intrathecal injections of galanin and its antiserum affect nociceptive response of rat to mechanical, but not thermal, stimuli. *Pain*, 1991, 44, 321-324.

Kutscha-Lissberg, F; Hebler, U; Muhr, G; Köller, M. Linezolid penetration into bone and joint tissues infected with methicillin-resistant staphylococci. *Antimicrob Agents Chemother*, 2003, 47, 3964-3966.

Kwok, BH; Koh, B; Ndubuisi, MI; Elofsson, M; Crews, CM . The anti-inflammatory natural product parthenolide from the medicinal herb Feverfew directly binds to and inhibits IkappaB kinase. *Chem. Biol.*, 2001, 8, 759-766.

Laird, JM; Carter, AJ; Grauert, M; Cervero F. Analgesic activity of a novel use-dependent sodium channel blocker, crobenetine, in mono-arthritic rats. *Br J Pharmacol*, 2001, 134, 1742-1748.

Lantz, RC; Chen, GJ; Sarihan, M; Sólyom, AM; Jolad, SD; Timmermann, BN. The effect of extracts from ginger rhizome on inflammatory mediator production. *Phytomedicine*, 2007, 14, 123-128.

Largo, R; Alvarez-Soria, MA; Díez-Ortego, I; Calvo, E; Sánchez-Pernaute, O; Egido, J; Herrero-Beaumont, G. Glucosamine inhibits IL-1beta-induced NFkappaB activation in human osteoarthritic chondrocytes. *Osteoarthritis Cartilage*, 2003, 11, 290-298.

Lascelles, BD; Gaynor, JS; Smith, ES; Roe, SC; Marcellin-Little, DJ; Davidson, G; Boland, E; Carr, J. Amantadine in a multimodal analgesic regimen for alleviation of refractory osteoarthritis pain in dogs. *J Vet Intern Med*, 2008, 22, 53-59.

Lautenschlager J. Present state of medication therapy in fibromyalgia syndrome. *Scand. J. Rheumatol (Suppl)*, 2000, 113, 32-36.

Leadbetter,W. Soft tissue athletic injuries. In: Fu FH, (Ed): *Sports Injuries: Mechanisms, Prevention, Treatment*. Baltimore: Williams and Wilkins; 1994; 736-737.

LeBars, D; Dickenson, AH; Besson, JM. Diffuse noxious inhibitory controls. Part I: effects on dorsal horn convergent neurones in the rat; Part II: lack of effect on nonconvergent neurones, supraspinal involvement and theoretical implications. *Pain*, 1979, 6, 283-327.

Lecomte, A; Costa, JP. Harpagophytum dans Parthrose Etudes en double insu contre placebo. *Le Magazine* 1992, 15, 27-30.

Lee, HM; Weinstein, JN; Meller, ST; Hayshi, N; Spratt, K; Gebhart, GF. The role of steroids and their effects on phospholipase A2: an animal model of radiculopathy. *Spine*, 1998, 23, 1191-1196.

Lee YW, Yaksh, TL. Pharmacology of the spinal adenosine receptor which mediates the antiallodynic action of intrathecal adenosine agonists. *J. Pharmacol Exp. Ther*, 1996, 277, 1642–1648.

Lembeck, F; Folkers, K; Donnerer, J. Analgesic effect of antagonists ofsubstance P. *Biochem Biophys Res Commun*, 1981, 103, 1318-1321.

Leslie, TA; Emson, PC; Dowd, PM; Woolf, CJ. Nerve-growth factor contributes to the upregulation of GAP-43 and preprotachykinin A mRNA in primary sensory neurons following peripheral inflammation. *Neuroscience*, 1995, 67, 753–761.

Levanthal, LJ; Boyce, EG; Zurier, RB. Treatment of rheumatoid arthritis with black current seed oil. *Br J Rheumatol*, 1994, 33, 847-852.

Levine, JD; Fields, HL; Basbaum, AI. Peptides and the primary afferent nociceptor. *J Neurosci*, 1993, 13, 2273-2286.

Levine, JD; Taiwo, YO. Involvement of the mu-opiate receptor in peripheral analgesia. *Neuroscience*, 1989, 32, 571-575.

Lew, DP; Waldvogel, FA. Osteomyelitis. *N Engl J Med*, 1997, 336, 999-1007.

Lin, EL; Lieu, V; Halevi, L; Shamie, AN; Wang, JC. Cervical epidural steroid injections for symptomatic disc herniations. *J Spinal Disord Tech*, 2006, 19, 183-186.

Lind, G; Schechtmann, G; Winter, J; Linderoth, B. Drug-enhanced spinal stimulation for pain: a new strategy. *Acta Neurochir Suppl*, 2007, 97(Pt 1), 57-63.

Liu, HX; Hökfelt, T. The participation of galanin in pain processing at the spinal level. *Trends Pharmacol Sci,* 2002, 23, 468-474.

Liu, H; Hökfelt, T. Effect of intrathecal galanin and its putative antagonist M35 on pain behavior in a neuropathic pain model. *Brain Res*, 2000, 886(1-2), 67-72.

Lott-Duarte, AH; Dourado, L; Tostes, M; Nascimento-Carvalho, CM. Extensive spondylodiscitis with epidural abscess causing fever and lower limbs pain in a child with sickle cell disease. *J Pediatr Hematol Oncol,* 2008, 30, 70-72.

Loubser, PG; Akman, NM. Effects of intrathecal baclofen on chronic spinal cord injury pain. *J Pain Symptom Manage*, 1996, 12, 241-247.

Lovering, AM; Walsh, TR; Bannister, GC; MacGowan, AP. The penetration of ceftriaxone and cefamandole into bone, fat and haematoma and relevance of serum protein binding to their penetration into bone. *J Antimicrob Chemother*, 2001, 47, 483-486.

Lovering, AM; Zhang, J; Bannister, GC; Lankester, BJ; Brown, JH; Narendra, G; MacGowan, AP. Penetration of linezolid into bone, fat, muscle and haematoma of patients undergoing routine hip replacement. *J Antimicrob Chemother*, 2002, 50, 73-77.

Lundin, A; Manguson, A; Axelsson, K; Nilson, O; Samuelsson, L. Corticosteroids preoperatively diminishes damage to the C-fibers in microscopic lumbar disc surgery. *Spine*, 2005, 30, 2362-2367.

Lynch, ME; Clark, AJ; Sawynok, J; Sullivan, MJ (a). Topical 2% amitriptyline and 1% ketamine in neuropathic pain syndromes: a randomized, double-blind, placebo-controlled trial. *Anesthesiology*, 2005,103,140-146.

Lynch, ME; Clark, AJ; Sawynok, J; Sullivan, MJ (b). Topical amitriptyline and ketamine in neuropathic pain syndromes: an open-label study. *J Pain*, 2005, 6, 644-649.

Ma, K; Jiang, W; Zhou, Q; Du, DP. The efficacy of oxycodone for management of acute pain episodes in chronic neck pain patients. *Int J Clin Pract*, 2007, 62, 241-247.

MacLeod, CM; Bartley, EA; Galante, JO; Friedhoff, LT; Dhruv, R. Aztreonam penetration into synovial fluid and bone. *Antimicrob Agents Chemother*, 1986, 29, 710-712.

Mader, JT; Adams, K; Morrison, L. Comparative evaluation of cefazolin and clindamycin in the treatment of experimental Staphylococcus aureus osteomyelitis in rabbits. *Antimicrob Agents Chemother*, 1989, 33, 1760-1764.

Madhusudan, S; Muthuramalingam, SR; Braybrooke, JP; Wilner, S; Kaur, K; Han, C; Hoare, S; Balkwill, F; Ganesan, TS. Study of etanercept, a tumor necrosis factor-alpha inhibitor, in recurrent ovarian cancer. *J Clin Oncol*, 2005, 23, 5950-5959.

Mahwold, ML; Singh, JA, Majeski, P. Opioid use by patients in an orthopedics spine clinc. *Arthritis Rheumatism*, 2005, 52, 312-321.

Makela, M; Heliovaara, M; Sievers, K; Impivaara, O; Knekt, P; Aromaa, A. Prevalence, determinants and consequences of chronic neck pain in Finland. *Am J Epidemiol*, 1991, 134, 1356-1367.

Makowska, A; Panfil, C; Ellrich, J. ATP induces sustained facilitation of craniofacial nociception through P2X receptors on neck muscle nociceptors in mice. *Cephalalgia*, 2006, 26, 697-706.

Malawski, SK; Lukawski, S. Pyogenic infection of the spine. *Clin. Orthop.*, 1991, 272, 58-66.

Malincarne, L; Ghebregzabher, M; Moretti, MV; Egidi, AM; Canovari, B; Tavolieri, G; Francisci, D; Cerulli, G; Baldelli F. Penetration of moxifloxacin into bone in patients undergoing total knee arthroplasty. *J Antimicrob Chemother*, 2006, 57, 950-954.

Malmberg, AB; Yaksh, TL (a). Hyperalgesia mediated by spinal glutamate or substance P receptor blocked by spinal cyclooxygenase inhibition. *Science*, 1992, 257(5074), 1276-1279.

Malmberg, AB; Yaksh, TL (b). Antinociceptive actions of spinal antisteroidal anti-inflammatory agents on the formalin test in the rat. *J Pharmacol Exp Ther*, 1992, 263, 136-146.

Manchikanti, L. Medicare in interventional pain management: a critical analysis. *Pain Physician*, 2006, 9, 171-198.

Manchikanti, L; Pampati, V; Damron, KS; McManus, CD; Jackson, SD; Barnhill, RC; Martin, JC (a). A randomized, prospective, double-blind, placebo-controlled evaluation of the effect of sedation on diagnostic validity of cervical facet joint pain. *Pain Physician*, 2004, 7, 301-309.

Manchikanti L, Boswell MV, Singh V, Pampati V, Damron KS, Beyer CD (b). Prevalence of facet joint pain in chronic spinal pain of cervical, thoracic, and lumbar regions. *BMC Musculoskelet Disord 2004*; 5: 15.

Manfredi, PL; Herskovitz, S; Folli, F; Pigazzi, A; Swerdlow, ML. Spinal epidural abscess: treatment options. *Eur Neurol*, 1998, 40, 58-60.

Mantyh, PW; DeMaster, E; Malhotra, A; Ghilardi, JR; Rogers, SD; Mantyh, CR; Liu, H; Basbaum, AI; Vigna, SR; Maggio, JE. Receptor endocytosis and dendrite reshaping in spinal neurons after somatosensory stimulation. *Science*, 1995, 268 (5217), 1629-1632.

Mantyh, PW; Rogers, SD; Honore, P; Allen, BJ; Ghilardi, JR; Li, J; Daughters, RS; Lappi, DA; Wiley, RG; Simone, DA. Inhibition of hyperalgesia by ablation of lamina I spinal neurons expressing the substance P receptor. *Science*, 1997, 278(5336), 275-279.

Mansour, A; Burke, S; Pavlic, RJ; Akil, H; Watson, SJ. Immunohistochemical localization of the cloned kappa 1 receptor in the rat CNS and pituitary. *Neuroscience*, 1996, 71, 671-690.

Mao, J. Translational pain research: bridging the gap between basic and clinical research. *Pain*, 2002, 97, 183–187.

Marchand, F; Tsantoulas, C; Singh, D; Grist, J; Clark, AK; Bradbury, EJ; McMahon, SB. Effects of Etanercept and Minocycline in a rat model of spinal cord injury. *Eur J Pain*, 2008, Oct 10.

Marcouiller, P; Pelletier, JP; Guévremont, M; Martel-Pelletier, J; Ranger, P; Laufer, S; Reboul, P. Leukotriene and prostaglandin synthesis pathways in osteoarthritic synovial membranes: regulating factors for interleukin 1beta synthesis. *J Rheumatol*, 2005, 32, 704-712.

Marienfeld, R; Neumann, M; Chuvpilo, S; Escher, C; Kneitz, B; Avots, A; Schimpl, A; Serfling, E. Cyclosporin A interferes with inducible degradation of NF-kB inhibitors but not with the processing of p105/NF-kB1 in T cells. *Eur J Immunol* 1997, 27, 1601-1609

Marroni, M; Tinca, M; Belfiori, B; Altobelli, G; Malincarne, L; Papili, R; Stagni, G. Nosocomial spondylodiskitis with epidural abscess and liquoral fistula cured with quinupristin/dalfopristin and linezolid. *Infez Med*, 2006, 14, 99-101.

Martin, RJ; Yuan, HA. Neurosurgical care of spinal epidural, subdural, and intramedullary abscesses and arachnoiditis. *Orthop Clin. North Am*, 1996, 27, 125-136.

Martin, TJ; Eisenach, JC; Misler, J; Childers, SR. Chronic activation of spinal adenosine A1 receptors results in hypersensitivity. *Neuroreport,* 2006, 17, 1619-1622.

Martinez, JH; Mondragon, CE; Céspedes, A. An evaluation of the antiinflammatory effects of intraarticular synthetic β-endorphin in the canine model. *Anesth Analg*, 1996, 82, 177-181.

Matsuki, A. Nothing new under the sun—a Japanese pioneer in the clinical use of intrathecal morphine. *Anesthesiology* 1983, 58, 289-290.

McCarthy, GM; Kenny, D. Dietary fish oil and rheumatic diseases. *Semin Arthritis Rheum*, 1992, 21, 368-375.

McCarthy, DJ; Csuka, M; McCarthy, G; Trotter, D. Treatment of pain due to fibromyalgia with topical capsaicin: a pilot study. *Semin Arthritis Rheum*, 1994, 23(suppl 3), 41-47.

McCleane, GJ (a). Topical doxepin hydrochloride reduces neuropathic pain: a randomized, double-blind, placebo controlled study. *Pain Clin*, 2000, 12, 47–50.

McCleane, GJ (b). Topical application of doxepin hydrochloride, capsaicin and a combination of both produces analgesia in chronic human neuropathic pain: a randomized, double-blind, placebo-controlled study. *Br J Clin Pharmacol*, 2000, 49, 574–579.

McCormack K. The spinal action of nonsteroidal anti-inflammatory drugs and the dissociation between their anti-inflammatory and analgesic effects. *Drugs* 1994, 47(Suppl 5), 28-45; Discussion 46-47.

McCormack, K; Kidd, BL; Morris, V. Assay of topically administered ibuprofen using a model of post-injury hypersensitivity. A randomised, double-blind, placebo-controlled study. *Eur J Clin Pharmacol*, 2000, 56(6-7), 459-462.

McDougall, JJ; Hanesch, U; Pawlak, M; Schmidt, RF. Participation of NK1 receptors in nociceptin-induced modulation of rat knee joint mechanosensitivity. *Exp Brain Res*, 2001, 137, 249-253.

McDougall, JJ; Watkins, L; Li, Z .Vasoactive intestinal peptide (VIP) is a modulator of joint pain in a rat model of osteoarthritis. *Pain*, 2006, 123(1-2), 98-105.

McHenry, MC; Easley, KA; Locker, GA. Vertebral osteomyelitis: long-term outcome for 253 patients from 7 Cleveland-area hospitals. *Clin Infect Dis*, 2002, 34, 1342-1350.

McMillan, A; Nolan, A; Kelly, P. The efficacy of dry needling and procaine in the treatment of myofascial pain in the jaw muscles. *J Orof Pain*, 1997, 11, 307-314.

Merskey, H; Watson, GD. The lateralisation of pain. *Pain*, 1979, 7, 271-280.

Michael, GJ; Averill, S; Nitkunan, A; Rattray, M; Bennett, DL; Yan, Q; Priestley, JV. Nerve growth factor treatment increases brain-derived neurotrophic factor selectively in TrkA-expressing dorsal root ganglion cells and in their central terminations within the spinal cord. *J Neurosci*, 1997, 17, 8476–8490.

Miljanich, GP; Ramachandran, J. Antagonists of neuronal calcium channels: structure, function, and therapeutic implications. *Annu Rev Pharmacol Toxicol*. 1995, 35, 707-734.

Mironer, EY; Haasis, JC; Chapple, I; Brown, C; Satterthwaite, JR. Efficacy and safety of intrathecal opioid/bupivacaine mixture in chronic nonmalignant pain: A double blind, randomized, crossover, multicenter study by the National Forum of Independent Pain Clinicians (NFIPC). *Neuromodulation*, 2002, 5, 208-213.

Mollenholt, P; Post, C; Rawal, N; Freedman, J; Hökfelt, T; Paulsson, I. Antinociceptive and 'neurotoxic' actions of somatostatin in rat spinal cord after intrathecal administration. *Pain*, 1988, 32, 95-105.

Molloy, RE; Benzon, HT. Interlaminar epidural steroid injections for lumbosacral radiculopathy. In: Benzon HT, Raja SN, Molloy RE, Liu SS, Fishman SM, editors. *Essentials of Pain Medicine and Regional Anesthesia*. Philadelphia, PA: Elsevier Churchill Livingstone; 2005; 331–340.

Moore, RA; Tramèr, MR; Carroll, D; Wiffen, PJ; McQuay, HJ. Quantitative systematic review of topically applied non-steroidal anti-inflammatory drugs. *BMJ,* 1998, 316(7128), 333-338.

Moriya, M; Kimura, T;Yamamoto,Y; Abe, K; Sakoda, S. Successful treatment of cervical spinal epidural abscess without surgery. *Intern Med*, 2005, 44, 1110.

Morton, CR; Hutichson, WD; Hendry, IA. Release of immunoreactive somatostatin in the spinal dorsal horn of the cat. *Neuropeptides*, 1988, 12, 189-197.

Morton, CR; Hutichson, WD. Release of sensory neuropeptides in the spinal cord: Studies with calcitonin gene related peptide and galanin. *Neuroscience*, 1989, 31, 807-815.

Muller, JL; Clauson, KA. Pharmaceutical considerations of common herbal medicine. *Am J Manag Care*, 1997, 3, 1753-1770.

Muller, R; Giles, LG. Long-term follow-up of a randomized clinical trial assessing the efficacy of medication, acupuncture, and spinal manipulation for chronic mechanical spinal pain syndromes. *J Manipulative Physiol Ther*, 2005, 28, 3-11.

Müller, J; Kemmler, G; Wissel, J; Schneider, A; Voller, B; Grossmann, J; Diez, J; Homann, N; Wenning, GK; Schnider, P; Poewe, W. The impact of blepharospasm and cervical dystonia on health-related quality of life and depression. *J Neurol*, 2002, 249, 842-846.

Murga, G; Samsó, E; Valles, J; Casanovas, P; Puig, MM. The effect of clonidine on intra-operative requirements of fentanyl during combined epidural/general anaesthesia. *Anaesthesia*, 1994, 49, 999-1002.

Muro, K; O'shaughnessy, B; Ganju, A. Infarction of the cervical spinal cord following multilevel transforaminal epidural steroid injection: case report and review of the literature. *J Spinal Cord Med*, 2007, 30, 385–388.

Naguib, M; Yaksh, TL. Antinociceptive effects of spinal cholinesterase inhibition and isobolographica. *Anesthesiology*, 1994, 80, 1338-1348.

Nagy, JI; Van Der Kooy, D. Effects on neonatal capsaicin treatment on nociceptive thresholds in the rat. *J Neurosci*, 1983, 3, 1145-1150.

Nakagawa, T; Wakamatsu, K; Zhang, N; Maeda, S; Minami, M; Satoh, M; Kaneko, S. Intrathecal administration of ATP produces long-lasting allodynia in rats: differential mechanisms in the phase of the induction and maintenance. *Neuroscience*, 2007,147, 445-455.

Najm, WI; Reinsch, S; Hoehler F, Tobis, JS; Harvey, PW. S-Adenosylmethionine (SAMe) versus celecoxibfor the treatment of osteoarthritissymptoms: A double-blind-cross-over trial. *BMC Musculoskeletal Disorders*, 2004, 5, 6.

Nallu, R; Radhakrishnan, R. Spinal release of acetylcholine in response to morphine. *J Pain*, 2007, 8, S19.

Neame, R; Zhang, W; Doherty, M. A historic issue of the Annals: three papers examine paracetamol in osteoarthritis. *Ann Rheum Dis* 2004, 63, 897-900.

Neugebauer, V; Rümenapp, P; Schaible, HG. Calcitonin gene-related peptide is involved in the spinal processing of mechanosensory input from the rat's knee joint and in the generation and maintenance of hyperexcitability of dorsal horn-neurons during development of acute inflammation. *Neuroscience*, 1996, 71, 1095-1109.

Nicholas, P; Meyers, BR; Levy, RN; Hirschman, SZ. Concentration of clindamycin in human bone. *Antimicrob Agents Chemother*, 1975, 8, 220-221.

Norimoto, M; Ohtori, S; Yamashita, M; Inoue, G; Yamauchi, K; Koshi, T; Suzuki, M; Orita, S; Eguchi, Y; Sugiura, A; Ochiai, N; Takaso, M; Takahashi, K. Direct application of the TNF-alpha inhibitor, etanercept, does not affect CGRP expression and phenotypic change of DRG neurons following application of nucleus pulposus onto injured sciatic nerves in rats. *Spine,* 2008, 33, 2403-2408.

Nozaki-Taguchi, N; Yaksh, TL. Characterization of the antihyperalgesic action of a novel peripheral mu-opioid receptor agonist--loperamide. *Anesthesiology*, 1999, 90, 225-234.

Oatway, M; Reid, A; Sawynok, J; Peripheral antihyperalgesic and analgesic actions of ketamine and amitriptyline in a model of mild thermal injury in the rat. *Anesth Analg*, 2003, 97,168-173.

Ojala,T; Arokoski, P; Partanen, J. The effect of small doses of botulinium toxin on a neck shoulder myofacial pain syndrome. A double blind randomized, and controlled crossover trial. *Clin J Pain*, 2006, 22, 90-96.

Oku, R; Satoh, M; Fujii, N; Otaka, A; Yajima, H; Takagi, H. calcitonon gene related peptide promotes mechanical nociception by potentiating releaseof substance P from the spinal dorsal horn in rats. *Brain Res*, 1987, 403, 350-354.

Olesen, J; Diener, H-C; Husstedt, IW; Godasby, PJ; Hall, D; Meier, U; Pollentier, S; Lesko, LM. Calcitonin gene-related peptide (CGRP) receptor antagonist BIBN4096BS for the acute treatment of migraine. *N Engl J Med*, 2004, 350, 1104–1110.

Olivera, B; Gray, WR; Zeikus, R; McIntosh, JM; Varga, J; Rivier, J;, deSantos, V; Cruz, LJ. Peptide neurotoxins from fish-hunting cone snails. *Science*, 1985, 230,1338-1343.

Olivera, BM; Cruz, LJ; de Santos, V; LeCheminant, GW;Griffin, D; Zeikus, R; McIntosh, JM; Galyean, R; Varga, J; Gray, WR; et al. Neuronal calcium channel antagonists. Discrimination between calcium channel subtypes using omega-conotoxin from Conus magus venom. *Biochemistry*, 1987, 26, 2086-2090.

Ossipov, MH; Bazov, I; Gardell, LR; Kowal, J; Yakovleva, T; Usynin, I; Ekström, TJ; Porreca, F; Bakalkin, G. Control of chronic pain by the ubiquitin proteasome system in the spinal cord. *J Neurosci*, 2007, 27, 8226-8237.

Osti, OL; Fraser, RD; Vernon-Roberts, B. Discitis after discography. The role of prophylactic antibiotics. *J. Bone Joint Surg Br*, 1990, 72, 271-274.

Paliwal, S; Sundaram, J; Mitragotri, S. Induction of cancer-specific cytotoxicity towards human prostate and skin cells using quercetin and ultrasound. *Br J Cancer*, 2005, 92, 499-502.

Pan, HL; Khan, GM; Alloway, KD; Chen, SR. Resiniferatoxin induces paradoxical changes in thermal and mechanical sensitivities in rats: mechanism of action. *J Neurosci*, 2003, 23, 2911–2919.

Paoloni, JA; Appleyard, RC; Nelson, J; Murrell, GA. Topical Nitric Oxide Application in the Treatment of Chronic Extensor Tendinosis at the Elbow. A Randomized, Double-Blinded, Placebo-Controlled Clinical Trial. *The American Journal of Sports Medicine*, 2003, 31, 915-920.

Park, JY; Jun, IG. The interaction of gabapentin and N6-(2-phenylisopropyl)-adenosine R-(-)isomer (R-PIA) on mechanical allodynia in rats with a spinal nerve ligation. *J Korean Med Sci,* 2008, 23, 678-684.

Paulose-Ram, R; Hirsch, R; Dillon, C; Gu, Q. Frequent monthly use of selected non-prescription and prescription non-narcotic analgesics among U.S. adults. *Pharmacoepidemiol Drug Saf*, 2005, 14, 257-266.

Pavelka, K; Gatterova, J; Olejarova, M; Machacek, S; Giacovelli, G; Rovati, LC. Glucosamine sulfate use and delay of progression of knee osteoarthritis: a 3-year, randomized, placebo-controlled, double-blind study. *Arch Intern Med*, 2002, 162, 2113-2123.

Pederson, JL; Galle, TS; Kehlet, H. Peripheral analgesic effects of ketamine in acute inflammatory pain. *Anesthesiology,* 1998, 89, 58-66.

Penerai, AE; Massei, R; DeSilva, G; Sacerdote, P; Monza, G; mantegazza, P. Baclofen prolongs the analgesic effect of fentanyl in man. *British Journal of Anaesthesia* 1985, 57, 954-955.

Pert, CB; Snyder, S. Opiate receptor: Demonstration in nervous tissue. *Science*, 1973, 179, 1011-1014.

Pertwee, RG. Cannabinoid receptors and pain. *Prog Neurobiol*, 2001, 63, 569-611.

Picavet, HS; Schouten, JS: Musculoskeletal pain in the Netherlands: prevalences, consequences and risk groups, the DMC(3)-study. *Pain*, 2003, 102(1–2), 167-178.

Pincus, T; Koch, G; Lei, H; Mangal, B; Sokka, T; Moskowitz, R; Wolfe, F; Gibofsky, A; Simon,L; Zlotnick, S; Fort, JG. Patient Preference for Placebo, Acetaminophen (paracetamol) or Celecoxib Efficacy Studies (PACES): two randomised, double blind, placebo controlled, crossover clinical trials in patients with knee or hip osteoarthritis. *Ann Rheum Dis*, 2004, 63, 931-939.

Pini, LA; Sandrini, M; Vitale, G. The antinociceptive action of paracetamol is associated with changes in the serotonergic system in the rat brain. *Eur J Pharmacol*, 1996, 308, 31-40.

Podichetty,VK. The aging spine: the role of inflammatory mediators in intervertebral disc degeneration. *Cell Mol Biol*, 2007, 53, 4-18.

Pohl, M; Lombard, MC; Bourgoin, S; Carayon, A; Benoliel, JJ; Mauborgne, A; Besson, JM; Cesselin, F. Opioid control of the in vitro release of calcitonin gene-related peptide from primary afferent fibres projecting in the rat cervical cord. *Neuropeptides,* 1989, 14, 151–159.

Post, C; Alari, L; Hökfelt, T. Intrathecal galanin increases the latency in the tail-flick and hot-plate test in mouse. *Acta Physiol Scand*, 1988, 132, 583-584.

Prado, WA; Dias, TB. Postoperative Analgesia Induced by Intrathecal Neostigmine or Bethanechol in Rats. *Clin Exp Pharmacol Physiol,* 2008 Nov 28.

Qerama, E; Fugisang-Frederiksen, A; Kasch , H; Bach, FW; Jensen, TS. A double blind controlled study of botulinum toxin A in chronic myofacial pain. *Neurology*, 2006, 67, 241-245.

Qinyang, W; Hultenby, K; Adlan, E; Lindgren, JU. Galanin in adjuvant arthritis in the rat. *J Rheumatol*, 2004, 31, 302-307.

Radhakrishnan, V; Henry, JL. Electrophysiology of neuropeptides in the sensory spinal cord. *Prog Brain Res* , 1995, 104, 175-195.

Rahme, E; Barkun, A; Nedjar, H; Gaugris, S; Watson, D. Hospitalizations for upper and lower GI events associated with traditional NSAIDs and acetaminophen among the elderly in Quebec, Canada. *Am J Gastroenterol*, 2008, 103, 872-882.

Rao, SG. The neuropharmacology of centrally-acting analgesic medications in fibromyalgia. *Rheum Dis Clin North Am*, 2002, 28, 235-259.

Recommendations for the medical management of osteoarthritis of the hip and knee: 2000 update. American College of Rheumatology Subcommittee on Osteoarthritis Guidelines. *Arthritis Rheum*, 2000, 43, 1905-1915.

Reeves, KD. Prolotherapy: Present and Future Applications in Soft-Tissue Pain and Disability. Injection Techniques: Principles and Practice. *Physical Medicine and Rehabilitation Clinics of North America*, 1995, 4, 917-923.

Reeves, KD. Prolotherapy: Basic Science, Clinical Studies, and Technique. In: Lennard TA (Ed): *Pain Procedures in Clinical Practice*, 2nd edition. Philadelphia; Hanley and Belfus; 2000; 172-190.

Reginster, JY; Deroisy, R; Rovati, LC; Lee, RL; Lejeune, E; Bruyere, O; Giacovelli, G; Henrotin, Y; Dacre, JE; Gossett, C. Long-term effects of glucosamine sulphate on osteoarthritis progression: a randomised, placebo-controlled clinical trial. *Lancet*, 2001, 357, 251-256.

Reynolds, IJ; Miller, RJ. Tricyclic antidepressants block N-methyl-D-aspartate receptors: similarities to the action of zinc. *Br J Pharmacol*, 1988, 95, 95–102.

Rezai, M; Côté, P; Cassidy, JD; Carroll, L. The association between prevalent neck pain and health-related quality of life: a cross-sectional analysis. *Eur Spine J*, 2008 Nov 20.

Rhoten, RLP; Murphy, MA; Kalfas, IH; Hahn, JF; Washington, JA. Antibiotic penetration into cervical discs. *Neurosurgery*, 1995, 37, 418-421.

Richardson, BP; Engel, G; Donatsch, P; Stadler, PA. Identification of serotonin M-receptor subtypes and their specific blockade by a new class of drugs. *Nature*, 1985, 316 (6024), 126-131.

Richy, F; Bruyere, O; Ethgen, O; Cucherat, M; Henrotin, Y; Reginster, J-Y. Structural and symptomatic efficacy of glucosamine and chondroitin in knee osteoarthritis. A comprehensive meta-analysis. *Arch Intern Med*, 2003, 163, 1514-1522.

Rimmelé, T; Boselli, E; Breilh, D; Djabarouti, S; Bel, JC; Guyot, R; Saux, MC; Allaouchiche, B. Diffusion of levofloxacin into bone and synovial tissues. *J Antimicrob Chemother*, 2004; 53: 533-535.

Rosomoff, HL; Fishbain, DA; Goldberg, M; Santana, R; Rosomoff, RS. Physical findings in patients with chronic intractable benign pain of the neck and/or back. *Pain*, 1989, 37, 279-287.

Rowlingson, JC; Kirschenbaum, LP. Epidural analgesic techniques in the management of cervical pain. *Anesth Analg*, 1986, 65, 938-942.

Ruan, X. Drug-related side effects of long-term intrathecal morphine therapy: A focused review. *Pain Physician*, 2007, 10, 357-366.

Rueff, A; Dray, A. Pharmacological characterization of the effects of 5-hydroxytryptamine and different prostaglandins on peripheral sensory neurons in vitro. *Agents Actions*, 1993, C13-15.

Ryöppy, S; Jääskeläinen, J; Rapola, J; Alberty, A. Nonspecific diskitis in children. A nonmicrobial disease? *Clin Orthop*, 1993, 297, 95-99.

Salonen, MA; Kanto, JH; Maze, M. Clinical interactions with alpha-2-adrenergic agonists in anesthetic practice. *J Clin Anesth*, 1992, 4, 164-172.

Sang, C; Jenkins, K; Wang, K; Sarin, A; Coccoli, S. Fosphenytoin relieves neuropathic pain following spinal cord injury. *Program and abstracts of the 25th Annual Scientific Meeting of the American Pain Society*; May 3-6, 2006; San Antonio, Texas. Poster 692.

Sano, T; Sakurai, M; Dohi, S; Oyama,A; Murota, K; Sugiyama, H; Miura, Y; Kusuoka, K; Kurata, K. Investigation of meropenem levels in the human bone marrow blood, bone, joint fluid and joint tissues. *Jpn J Antibiot*, 1993, 46,159-163.

Sapico, FL: Microbiology and antimicrobial therapy of spinal infections. *Orthop Clin North Am*, 1996, 27, 9-13.

Sapico, FL; Montgomerie, JZ. Pyogenic vertebral osteomyelitis: re port of nine cases and review of the literature. *Rev Infect Dis*, 1979, 1,754-776.

Sastravaha, G; Gassman, G; Sangtherapitikul, P; Grimm, WD. Adjunctive periodontal therapy with Centella asiatica and Punica granatum extracts in supportive periodontal therapy. *J Int Acad Periodontl*, 2005, 7, 70-79.

Sawynok J, Sweeney MI. The role of purines in nociception. *Neuroscience*, 1989, 32, 557–569.

Schellingerhout, JM; Verhagen, AP; Heymans, MW; Pool, JJ; Vonk, F; Koes, BW; de Vet, HC. Which subgroups of patients with non-specific neck pain are more likely to benefit from spinal manipulation therapy, physiotherapy, or usual care? *Pain*, 2008, Sep 4.

Schimmer, RC; Jeanneret, C; Nunley, PD; Jeanneret, B. Osteomyelitis of the cervical spine: a potentially dramatic disease. *J Spinal Disord Tech*, 2002, 15, 110-117.

Schreiber, AL; Formal, CS. Spinal cord infarction secondary to cocaine use. *Am J Phys Med Rehabil*, 2007, 86, 158-160.

Schurman, DJ; Burton, DS; Kajiyama, G. Cefoxitin antibiotic concentration in bone and synovial fluid. *Clin. Orthop Relat Res.*, 1982, 168, 64-68.

Schofferman, J. Long-term use of opioid analgesics for the treatment of chronic pain of nonmalignant origin. *J Pain Symptom Manage*, 1993, 8, 279-288.

Scuderi, GJ; Greenberg, SS; Banovac, K; Martinez, OV; Eismont, FJ. Penetration of glycopeptide antibiotics in nucleus pulposus. *Spine*, 1993, 14, 2039-2042

See, S; Ginsburg, R. Choosing a skeletal muscle relaxant. *Am Fam Physician*, 2008, 78, 365-370.

Serhan, CN. Lipoxins and aspirin-triggered 15-epi-lipoxins are the first lipid mediators of endogenous anti-inflammation and resolution. *Prostaglandins Leukot Essent Fatty Acids*, 2005, 73(3-4), 141-162.

Serhan, CN. Resolution phase of inflammation: novel endogenous anti-inflammatory and proresolving lipid mediators and pathways. *Annu Rev Immunol*, 2007, 25, 101–137.

Serhan, CN; Chiang, N; Van Dyke, TE. Resolving inflammation: dual anti-inflammatory and pro-resolution lipid mediators. *Nat Rev Immunol*, 2008, 8, 349-361.

Serhan, CN; Hamberg, M; Samuelsson, B. Lipoxins: novel series of biologically active compounds formed from arachidonic acid in human leukocytes. *Proc Natl Acad Sci USA*, 1984, 81, 5335-5339.

Serhan, CN; Hong, S; Gronert, K; Colgan, SP; Devchand, PR; Mirick, G; Moussignac, RL. Resolvins: a family of bioactive products of omega-3 fatty acid transformation circuits initiated by aspirin treatment that counter proinflammation signals. *J Exp Med*, 2002, 196, 1025-1037.

Serhan, C N; Savill, J. Resolution of inflammation: the beginning programs the end. *Nature Immunol*, 2005, 6, 1191–1197.

Sekiguchi, M; Shirasaka, M; Konno, S-I; Kikuchi, S. Analgesic effect of percutaneously absorbed non-steroidal anti-inflammatory drugs: an experimental study in a rat acute inflammation model. *BMC Muscloskeletal Disoredrs*, 2008, 9, 15.

Sharma, S; Chopra, K; Kulkarni, SK . Effect of insulin and its combination with resveratrol or curcumin in attenuation of diabetic neuropathic pain: participation of nitric oxide and TNF-alpha. *Phytother Res*, 2007, 147, 155-163.

Shen, CL; Hong, KJ; Kim, SW. Comparative effects of ginger root (Zingiber officinale Rosc.) on the production of inflammatory mediators in normal and osteoarthrotic sow chondrocytes. *J Med Food*, 2005, 8, 149-153.

Sherman, KJ; Cherkin, DC; Erro, J; Hrbek, A; Eisenberg, DM; Davis, RB. The diagnosis and treatment of chronic back pain by acupuncturist, chiropractors and massage therapists. *Clin J Pain*, 2006, 22, 227-234.

Shukla M, Gupta K, Rasheed Z, Khan KA, Haqqi TM. Bioavailable constituents/ metabolites of pomegranate (*Punica granatum* L) preferentially inhibit COX2 activity *ex vivo* and IL-1beta-induced PGE2 production in human chondrocytes *in vitro*. *Journal of Inflammation*, 2008, 5:9 doi:10.1186/1476-9255-5-9.

Siddall, PJ; Molloy, AR; Walker, S; Mather, LE; Rutkowski, SB; Cousins, MJ. The efficacy of intrathecal morphine and clonidine in the treatment of pain after spinal cord injury. *Anesth. Analg*, 2000, 91, 1493-1498.

Singh, G; Shetty, RR; Ramdass, MJ; Ravidass, MJ; Anilkumar, PG. Cervical osteomyelitis associated with intravenous drug use. *Emerg Med J*, 2006, 23, e16.

Sjölund, K-F; von Hejne, M; Hao, J-X. Intrathecal administration of the adenosine A1 receptor agonist R-phenylisopropyl adenosine reduces presumed pain behaviour in a rat model of central pain. *Neurosci Lett*, 1998, 243, 89–92.

Sodin-Semrl, S; Spagnolo, A; Barbaro, B; Varga, J; Fiore, S. Lipoxin A4 counteracts synergistic activation of human fibroblast-like synoviocytes. *Int J Immunopathol Pharmacol*, 2004, 17, 15-25.

Sodin-Semrl, S; Taddeo, B; Tseng, D; Varga, J; Fiore, S. Lipoxin A4 inhibits IL-1 beta-induced IL-6, IL-8, and matrix metalloproteinase-3 production in human synovial fibroblasts and enhances synthesis of tissue inhibitors of metalloproteinases. *J Immunol*, 2000, 164, 2660-2666.

Simone, DA; Alreja, M; LaMotte, RH. Psychophysical studies of the itch sensation and itchy skin ("alloknesis") produced by intracutaneous injection of histamine. *Somatosens Mot Res*, 1991, 8, 271-279.

Simons, DG; Travell, JG; Simons, LS. Travell and Simons' Myofascial Pain and Dysfunction: The Trigger Point Manual. 2nd edition. Baltimore: Williams and Wilkins; 2002.

Simons, DG: Fibrositis/fibromyalgia: a form of myofascial trigger points? *Am J Med*, 1986, 81, 93-98.

Singh, J; Budhiraja, S. Therapeutic potential of cannabinoid receptor ligands: current status. *Methods Find Exp Clin Pharmacol*, 2006, 28, 177-183.

Sist, T; Miner, M; Lema, M. Characteristics of postradical neck pain syndrome: a report of 25 cases. *J Pain Symptom Manage*, 1999, 18, 95-102.

Slipman, CW; Lipetz, JS; Jackson, HB; Rogers, DP; Vresilovic, EJ. Therapeutic selective nerve root block in the nonsurgical treatment of atraumatic cervical spondylotic radicular pain: a retrospective analysis with independent clinical review. *Arch Phys Med Rehabil*, 2000; 81:741–746.

Solomou, E; Maragkos, M; Kotsarini, C; Konstantinou, D; Maraziotis, T. Multiple spinal epidural abscesses extending to the whole spinal canal. *Magn Reson Imaging* 2004, 22, 747-750.

Staats, PS; Yearwood, T; Charapata, SG; Presley, RW; Wallace, MS; Byas-Smith, M; Fisher, R; Bryce, DA; Mangieri, EA; Luther, RR; Mayo, M; McGuire, D; Ellis, D. Intrathecal ziconotide in the treatment of refractory pain in patients with cancer or AIDS: A randomized controlled trial. *JAMA*, 2004, 291, 63-70.

Steen, AE; Reeh, PW; Geisslinger, G; Steen, KH. Plasma levels after peroral and topical ibuprofen and effects upon low pH-induced cutaneous and muscle pain. *Eur J Pain*, 2000, 4, 195-209.

Stein, C; Yassouridis A. Peripheral morphine analgesia. *Pain*, 1997; 71(2):119-121.

Suzuki, N; Hardebo, JE; Owman, C. Trigeminal fibre collaterals storing substance P and calcitonin gene-related peptide associate with ganglion cells containing choline acetyltransferase and vasoactive intestinal polypeptide in the sphenopalatine ganglion of the rat. An axon reflex modulating parasympathetic ganglionic activity? *Neuroscience*, 1989, 30, 595-604.

Svensson, CI; Zattoni, M; Serhan, CN. Lipoxins and aspirin-triggered lipoxins inhibit inflammatory pain processing. *J Exp Med*, 2007, 204, 245-252.

Sycha T, Kranz G, Auff E, Schnider P. Botulinum toxin in the treatment of rare head and neck pain syndromes: a systematic review of the literature. *J Neurol*, 2004, Feb, I19-30.

Szallasi, A; Blumberg, PM; Annicelli, LL; Krause, JE; Cortright, DN. The cloned rat vanilloid receptor VR1 mediates both R-type binding and C-type calcium response in dorsal root ganglion neurons. *Mol Pharmacol,* 1999, 56, 581–587.

Szallasi, A. Vanilloid receptor ligands: hopes and realities for the future. *Drugs Aging*, 2001, 18, 561–573.

Tai, CC; Want, S; Quraishi, NA; Batten, J; Kalra, J; Hughes, SPF. Antibiotic prophylaxis in surgery of the intervertebral disc: A comparison between gentamicin and cefuroxime. *J Bone Joint Surg [Br]*, 2002, 84-B, 1036-1039.

Taiwo YO, Levine JD. Kappa- and delta-opioids block sympathetically dependent hyperalgesia. *J Neurosci,* 1991, 11, 928-932.

Tal, M; Bennett, GJ. Dextrorphan relieves neuropathic heat-evoked hyperalgesia in the rat. *Neurosci Lett*, 1993, 141, 107–110.

Tandon, N; Vollmer, DG. Infections of the spine and spinal cord. In:Winn HR (ed). *Youmans Neurological Surgery*, edition 5. Philadelphia: Saunders; 2004; Vol 4; pp; 4363-4394.

Taricco, M; Pagliacci, MC; Telaro, E; Adone, R. Pharmacological interventions for spasticity following spinal cord injury: Results of a Cochrane systematic review. *Eura Medicophys*, 2006, 42, 5-15.

Tarsy, D. Comparison of acute- and delayed-onset posttraumatic cervical dystonia. *Mov Disord*, 1998, 13, 481-485.

Taylor, HH; Murphy, B. Altered sensorimotor integration with cervical spine manipulation. *J. Manipulative Physiol. Ther*, 2008, 31, 115-126.

Terenius, L. Characteristics of the "receptor" for narcotic analgesics in synaptic plasma membrane fractions from rat brain. *Acta Pharmacol Toxicol,* 1973, 33, 377-384.

Uchida, S; Hirai, K; Hatanaka, J; Hanato, J; Umegaki, K; Yamada, S. Antinociceptive Effects of St. John's Wort, Harpagophytum Procumbens Extract and Grape Seed Proanthocyanidins Extract in Mice. *Biol Pharm Bull*, 2008, 31, 240-245.

Tzchentke, TM; De Vry, J; Christoph, T et al. Tapentadol HCl: analgesic profile of a novel centrally active analgesic with dual mode of action in animal models of nociception, inflammatory and neuropathic pain. *Program and abstracts of the 25th Annual Scientific Meeting of the American Pain Society;* May 3-6, 2006; San Antonio, Texas. Poster 687.

Uhle, EI; Becker, R; Gatscher, S; Bertalanffy, H. Continuous intrathecal clonidine administration for the treatment of neuropathic pain. *Stereotact Funct Neurosurg*, 2000, 75, 167-175.

Urban, L; Thompson, SW; Dray, A. Modulation of spinal excitability: co-operation between neurokinin and excitatory amino acid neurotransmitters. *Trends Neurosci*, 1994, 17, 432-438.

Usha, PR; Naidu, MUR. Randomised, double-blind, parallel, placebo-controlled study of oral glucosamine, methylsulfonylmethane and their combination in osteoarthritis. *Clin Drug Invest*, 2004, 24, 353–363.

Vaile, JH; Davis, P. Topical NSAIDs for musculoskeletal conditions. A review of the literature. *Drugs*, 1998, 56, 783-799.

van der Velde, G; Hogg-Johnson, S; Bayoumi, AM; Cassidy, JD; Côté, P; Boyle, E; Llewellyn-Thomas, H; Chan, S; Subrata, P; Hoving, JL; Hurwitz, E; Bombardier, C; Krahn, M. Identifying the best treatment among common nonsurgical neck pain treatments: a decision analysis. *Spine*, 2008, 33(4 Suppl), S184-191.

van Dongen, RT; Crul, BJ; van Egmond, J. Intrathecal coadministration of bupivacaine diminishes morphine dose progression during long-term intrathecal infusion in cancer patients. *Clin J Pain*, 1999; 15:166-172.

van Hilten; BJ; van de Beek, WJ; Hoff, JI; Voormolen, JH; Delhaas, EM. Intrathecal baclofen for the treatment of dystonia in patients with reflex sympathetic dystrophy. *N Engl J Med*, 2000, 343,625-630.

Van Tulder, MW; Touray, T; Furla, AD; Solway, S; Bouter, LM. Muscle relaxants for non-specific low back pain. *Cochrane Database Syst Rev*, 2003, (2): CD004252.doi:10.1002/14651858:CD004252. PMID 12804507.

Vaught, JL. Substance P antagonists and analgesia: a review of the hypothesis. *Life Sci*, 1988, 43, 1419-1431.

Wagner, R; Myers, RR. Endoneurial injection of TNF-alpha produces neuropathic pain behaviors. *Neuroreport*, 1996, 7, 2897-2901.

Waldmann, R; Champigny, G; Bassilana, F; Heurteaux, C; Lazdunski, M. A proton-gated cation channel involved in acid-sensing. *Nature*, 1997, 386(6621), 173-177.

Walid, MS; Hyer, L; Ajjan, M; Barth, AC; Robinson, JS. Prevalence of opioid dependence in spine surgery and correlation with length stay. *J Opioid Manag*, 2007, 3, 127-128, 130-132.

Wallace, M; Yaksh, TL. Long term spinal analgesic delivery: A review of preclinical and clinical literature. *Reg Anesth Pain Med*, 2000, 25, 117-157.

Wallin, MK; Raak, RI. Quality of life in subgroups of individuals with whiplash associated disorders. *Eur J Pain*, 2008, 12, 842-849.

Walsh, AJ; O'neill, CW; Lotz, JC. Glucosamine HCl alters production of inflammatory mediators by rat intervertebral disc cells in vitro. *Spine J*, 2007, 7, 601-608.

Walters, R; Vernon-Roberts, B; Fraser, R; Moore, R. Therapeutic use of cephazolin to prevent complications of spine surgery. *Inflammopharmacology*, 2006, 14, 138-143.

Wang, SM; Kain, ZN; White, PF. Acupuncture analgesia: II. Clinical considerations. *Anesth Analg*, 2008,106, 611-621.

Warncke, T; Jorum, E; Stubhaug, A. Local treatment with N-methyl-D-aspartate receptor antagonist ketamine, inhibits development of secondary hyperalgesia in man by a peripheral action. *Neurosci Lett*, 1997, 227, 1-4.

Warner, TD; Mitchell, JA. Cyclooxygenase-3 (COX-3): filling in the gaps toward a COX continuum? *Proc Natl Acad Sci USA*, 2002, 99, 13371-13373.

Watson, CPN.Topical capsaicin as an adjuvant analgesic. *J Pain Symptom Manage*, 1994, 9, 425-433.

Watson, CP; Babul, N. Efficacy of oxycodone in neuropathic pain: a randomized trial in post-herpetic neuralgia. *Neurology*, 1998, 50, 1837-1841.

Weisman, H; Hagaman, C; Yaksh, TL; Lotz, M. Preliminaryfindings on the role of neuropeptide suppression bytopical agents in the managementof rheumatoid arthritis. *Seminars in Arthritisand Rheumatism*, 1994, 23 (suppl 3), 18-24.

Welch, SP; Stevens, DL. Antinociceptive activity of intrathecally administered cannabinoids alone, and in combination with morphine, in mice. *J Pharmacol Exp Ther*, 1992, 262, 10-18.

Welch, SP; Singha, AK; Dewey, WL. The antinociception produced by intrathecal morphine, calcium, A23187, U50, 488H, [D-Ala2, N-Me-Phe4, Glyol]enkephalin and [D-Pen2, D-Pen5]enkephalin after intrathecal administration of calcitonin gene-related peptide in mice. *J Pharmacol Exp Ther*, 1989, 251, 1–8.

Wenger, DR; Bobechko, WP; Gilday, DL. The spectrum of intervertebral disc-space infection in children. *J Bone Joint Surg Am*, 1978, 60, 100-108.

White, AR; Ernst, E. A systematic review of randomized controlled trials of acupuncture for neck pain. *Rheumatology*, 1999, 38, 143-147.

Wiech, K; Kiefer, RT; Töpfner, S; Preissl, H; Braun, C; Unertl, K; Flor, H; Birbaumer, N. A placebo-controlled randomized crossover trial of the N-methyl-D-aspartic acid receptor antagonist, memantine, in patients with chronic phantom limb pain. *Anesth Analg*, 2004, 98, 408-413.

Wood, R. Ketamine for pain in hospice patients. *Int J Pharm Compound.*, 2000, 4, 258–259.

Woolf ,CJ; Mannion, RJ. Neuropathic pain: Aetiology, symptoms, mechanisms and management. *Lancet*, 1999, 353, 1959-1964.

Wu, J. Anti-inflammatory ingredients. *J Drugs Dermatol*, 2008, 7(7 Suppl), S13-16.

Xu, XJ; Farkas-Szallasi, T; Lundberg, JM Hökfelt, T; Wiesenfeld-Hallin, Z; Szallasi, A . Effects of the capsaicin analogue resiniferatoxin on spinal nociceptive mechanisms in the rat: behavioural, electrophysiological and *in situ* hybridization studies. *Brain Res*, 1997, 752, 52–60.

Yaksh, TL. Behavioral and autonomic correlates of the tactile evoked allodynia produced by spinal glycine inhibition: effects of modulatory receptor systems and excitatory amino acid antagonists. *Pain*, 1989, 37, 111-123.

Yaksh, TL; Dirig, DM; Malmberg, AB. Mechanism of action of nonsteroidal anti-inflammatory drugs. *Cancer Invest*, 1998, 16, 509-527.

Yamauchi ,M; Asano, M; Watanabe, M; Iwasaki,S; Furuse, S; Namiki, A. Continuous dose ketamine improves the analgesic effects of fentanyl patient-controlled analgesia after cervical spine surgery. *Anesth Analg*, 2008, 107, 1041-1041.

Yanagisawa, M; Yagi, N; Otsuka, M; Yanaihara, C; Yanaihara, N. Inhibitory effects of galanin on the isolated spinal cord of the newborn rat. *Neurosci Lett*, 1986, 70, 278-282.

Yelland, MJ; Nikles, CJ; McNairn, N; Del Mar, CB; Schluter, PJ; Brown, RM. Celecoxib compared with sustained-release paracetamol for osteoarthritis: a series of n-of-1 trials. *Rheumatololgy* (Oxford), 2006, 46, 135-140.

Yu, LC; Lundeberg, S; An, H; Wang, FX; Lundeberg, T. Effects of intrathecal galanin on nociceptive responses in rats with mononeuropathy. *Life Sci*, 1999, 64, 1145-1153.

Zanella, JM; Burright, EN; Hildebrand, K; Hobot, C; Cox, M; Christoferson, L; McKay, WF. Effect of etanercept, a tumor necrosis factor-alpha inhibitor, on neuropathic pain in the rat chronic constriction injury model. *Spine*, 2008, 33, 227-234.

Zesiewicz, TA; Stamey, W; Sullivan, KL; Hauser, RA. Botulinum toxin A for the treatment of cervical dystonia. *Expert Opin Pharmacother*, 2004, 5, 2017-2024.

Zhang, W; Jones, A; Doherty, M. Does paracetamol (acetaminophen) reduce the pain of osteoarthritis? A meta-analysis of randomised controlled trials. *Ann Rheum Dis*, 2004, 63, 901-907.

Zhang, HM; Chen, SR; Cai, YQ; Richardson, TE; Driver, LC; Lopez-Berestein, G; Pan, HL. Signaling mechanisms mediating muscarinic enhancement of GABAERGIC synaptic transmission in the spinal cord. *Neuroscience*, 2008 Dec 7.

Zochodne, DW; Ho, LT. Sumatriptan blocks neurogenic inflammation in the peripheral nerve trunk. *Neurology*, 1994, 44, 161-163.

Zubrzycka, M; Janecka, A; KoziolKiewicz, W; Traczyk, WZ. Inhibition of tongue reflex in rats by tooth pulb stimulation during cerebral ventricle perfusion with (6-11) substance P analogs. *Brain Res*, 1997, 753, 128-132.

Zwart, JA; Dyb, G; Hagen, K; Svebak, S; Holmen, J. Analgesic use: a predictor of chronic pain and medication overuse headache: the Head-HUNT Study. *Neurology*, 2003, 61,160-164.

Zygmunt, PM; Petersson, J; Andersson, DA; Chuang, H; Sørgård, M; Di Marzo, V; Julius, D; Högestätt, ED . Vanilloid receptors on sensory nerves mediate the vasodilator action of anandamide. *Nature*, 1999, 400 (6743), 452- 457.

Index

A

acetaminophen, vii, 21, 22, 23, 83, 84, 104, 113
acetylcholine, 30, 38, 43, 101
acid, 3, 5, 7, 8, 10, 11, 14, 15, 17, 18, 19, 20, 21, 35, 47, 62, 64, 66, 68, 83, 107, 110, 111, 112
acidity, 16
action potential, 16
acupuncture, 55, 61, 72, 88, 89, 92, 101, 112
adalimumab, 36
adenosine, 5, 16, 38, 63, 77, 79, 96, 99, 103, 108
adenosine triphosphate, 63
adrenal gland, 67
adrenal glands, 67
adverse event, 63
afferent nerve, 8
age, 1, 25, 51, 71, 78
agonist, 24, 29, 32, 35, 38, 46, 47, 86, 102, 108
AIDS, 109
alcohol, 59
alcoholism, 53
allergic reaction, 42, 46
allergy, 42, 60
alternative medicine, 55
alters, 19, 111
amino acids, 5
anaerobic bacteria, 50, 81
analgesic, 6, 10, 18, 21, 22, 23, 24, 25, 26, 32, 33, 34, 35, 37, 38, 40, 41, 42, 43, 46, 55, 58, 64, 66, 69, 81, 83, 85, 92, 95, 99, 102, 103, 104, 105, 110, 111, 112, 113
analgesic agent, 85
anesthetics, 46
ankylosing spondylitis, 36, 81
anterior cruciate, 86
antibiotic, 52, 106
antibody, 31, 87
anti-inflammatories, 87
anti-inflammatory agents, 98
anti-inflammatory drugs, vii, 3, 22, 60, 64, 73, 85, 99, 113
antimicrobial therapy, 51, 106
antioxidant, 69
antipyretic, 22, 23, 65, 66, 83
arachnoiditis, 99
artery, 27, 45, 79, 81
arthritis, 9, 27, 44, 62, 63, 66, 68, 69, 77, 104
arthroscopy, 24, 86
articular cartilage, 79, 82
aspartate, 5, 33, 93, 94, 105, 111
assessment, 71, 72, 81, 92
asymptomatic, 32
ATP, 5, 9, 13, 19, 38, 63, 87, 97, 101

autoimmune disease, 36
axon terminals, 47

B

bacillus, 29
back pain, 1, 4, 25, 32, 34, 36, 37, 59, 61, 71, 72, 77, 78, 81, 83, 84, 85, 88, 90, 107, 111
bacteria, 49, 52
Beck Depression Inventory, 72
behavior, 6, 92, 96
beneficial effect, vii, 35
benign, 51, 105
binding, 24, 37, 47, 49, 97, 109
biofeedback, 57
biological activity, 30, 37
biologically active compounds, 107
biosynthesis, 17, 63, 84
blepharospasm, 30, 80, 101
blocks, 30, 37, 65, 82, 113
blood, 20, 32, 36, 39, 44, 50, 58, 106
blood flow, 58
blood pressure, 32
blood stream, 36
bone, 1, 49, 52, 59, 89, 95, 96, 97, 98, 102, 105, 106
bone marrow, 106
bones, 50, 58
brachial plexus, 79, 89
bradycardia, 32
bradykinin, 5, 7, 12, 18, 24, 57, 82
brain, 7, 10, 16, 24, 32, 35, 39, 46, 100, 104, 110
brain stem, 46
bronchial asthma, 39
burning, 27, 41

C

calcitonin, vii, 5, 6, 7, 9, 78, 86, 101, 104, 109, 112
calcium, 9, 11, 13, 27, 35, 38, 47, 58, 102, 109, 112
Canada, 104
cancer, 39, 40, 43, 46, 47, 103, 109, 111
candidates, 53
cannabinoids, 39, 112
cartilage, 37, 62, 64, 67, 82
cation, 16, 111
cefazolin, 49, 51, 53, 88, 97
cell, 13, 18, 37, 46, 59, 63, 65, 88
cell membranes, 63
central nervous system, 5, 6, 27, 33, 38, 56
cerebrospinal fluid, 12
cervical radiculopathy, 81, 94
cervical spondylosis, 25, 56, 89
channel blocker, 16, 34, 94, 95
channels, 9, 16, 38, 46, 47, 80
chemiluminescence, 81
chemokines, 15
chemotaxis, 14
children, 51, 81, 106, 112
cholinesterase, 38, 101
cholinesterase inhibitors, 39
chondrocyte, 90
chromosome, 7, 17
circulation, 21, 57
clinical symptoms, 73
clinical trials, 62, 87, 104
cluster headache, 28
CNS, 98
coagulopathy, 42
cocaine, 27, 106
cohort, 57, 72, 80
collateral damage, 15
combination therapy, 83
compensation, 72, 91
complexity, 75
compliance, 20, 93
complications, 42, 43, 45, 111
components, 72, 87
compounds, 15, 28, 58, 69
compression, 46, 57, 62
concentration, 9, 19, 47, 49, 106
conduction, 8, 28, 29, 94
connective tissue, 59, 67
control, 12, 25, 40, 56, 60, 63, 72, 82, 92, 104

Index

control group, 72
controlled trials, 41, 56, 61, 63, 78, 112, 113
cortical bone, 49, 92
corticosteroids, 44, 46, 79
coupling, 16
COX-2 enzyme, 14, 67
critical analysis, 98
cross-sectional study, 72
crystalline, 27, 28
cyclooxygenase, 22, 64, 68, 83, 98
cytochrome, 22
cytokines, 5, 13, 14, 15, 19, 36, 67
cytotoxicity, 103

D

debridement, 86
deficit, vii, 45, 53
degradation, 37, 48, 86, 99
delivery, 39, 41, 91, 111
dendrites, 47
Denmark, 93
depression, 56, 63, 72, 81, 101
derivatives, 83
dermis, 21
desensitization, 27
destruction, 6, 8, 26
diabetic neuropathy, 28, 34, 40
differentiation, 90
disability, 1, 56, 71, 72, 80, 84, 88, 90, 94
discitis, vii, 50, 51, 84, 103
discomfort, 41, 57
discs, 12, 51, 93, 105
disease activity, 37, 64
diskitis, 81, 106
disorder, 28, 29, 30, 46, 71, 72
dissociation, 99
distribution, 27
DNA, 36
docosahexaenoic acid, 15
dopamine, 81
dorsal horn, 5, 6, 7, 8, 10, 11, 19, 22, 33, 43, 86, 87, 88, 93, 95, 101, 102
double blind study, 32
drug abuse, 26, 53, 78, 81
drug use, 108
drugs, 17, 18, 26, 31, 32, 34, 36, 39, 44, 51, 52, 75, 82, 83, 89, 105
duration, 4, 30, 35, 40, 46, 56, 58, 72, 80
dystonia, 29, 30, 31, 35, 47, 73, 75, 80, 82, 84, 87, 101, 110, 111, 113

E

edema, 7
editors, 100
eicosapentaenoic acid, 15
elderly, 56, 88, 104
electromyography, 30
emboli, 45
embolization, 45
emotional experience, 3
encoding, 7, 78, 82
endorphins, 24, 55
endothelium, 7
England, 16, 79, 87
enkephalins, 7, 24
enzymes, 11, 18, 22
epidural abscess, 49, 50, 51, 53, 79, 85, 96, 98, 99, 101, 109
epinephrine, 89
erythrocyte sedimentation rate, 52
ESR, 52
etanercept, 36, 81, 89, 97, 102, 113
etiology, 11
Europe, 63
excitability, 9, 14, 110
excitation, 13, 29
exercise, 1, 3, 37, 60, 72, 73, 81, 93
extensor, 12, 31

F

false negative, 42
family, 8, 17, 27, 107
fatigue, 37, 64, 65
fatty acids, 15, 63, 85
FDA, 22, 30, 43, 46, 47
FDA approval, 22, 30

fever, 18, 22, 37, 96
fibers, 6, 8, 11, 24, 44, 89, 93, 97
fibroblasts, 15, 59, 77, 108
fibromyalgia, 1, 4, 34, 35, 57, 64, 65, 75, 82, 92, 95, 99, 104, 108
Finland, 97
first-generation cephalosporin, 49, 51
fish, 63, 99, 102
fish oil, 63, 99
fluid, 42, 50, 59, 106
free radicals, 13
fungal infection, 52
fusion, 26, 29, 36, 37, 86

G

ganglion, 6, 9, 10, 72, 87, 91, 100, 109
gel, 39
gender, 71, 72, 78
gene, vii, 5, 6, 7, 8, 9, 22, 78, 82, 86, 101, 102, 104, 109, 112
gene expression, 78, 82
generation, 10, 14, 58, 102
genes, 8
ginger, 95, 107
ginseng, 66, 67
glaucoma, 39
glutamate, 5, 24, 93, 98
glycine, 5, 11, 112
glycosaminoglycans, 61
groups, 41, 51, 104
growth, 14, 15, 51, 59, 87, 96, 100
growth factor, 14, 15, 59, 87, 96, 100

H

half-life, 36
headache, 1, 2, 12, 25, 42, 44, 60, 75, 92, 113
healing, 21, 58, 59, 68, 88
health, 4, 61, 71, 72, 81, 101, 105
heat, vii, 1, 23, 28, 41, 82, 109
hematoma, 45
hepatotoxicity, 22
herbal medicine, 64, 101
herniated, 2, 12, 42, 44
herniated nucleus pulposus, 42
heroin, 26, 87
hip, 62, 81, 97, 104, 105
hip replacement, 97
histamine, 5, 7, 13, 56, 69, 108
HIV infection, 53
hospitalization, 23
hospitals, 69, 100
hydrogen peroxide, 12
hydroxyl, 12
hyperhidrosis, 30
hypersensitivity, 4, 18, 38, 40, 99
hypothesis, 111

I

ibuprofen, 22, 36, 83, 99, 109
idiopathic, 42
IL-6, 5, 62, 67, 108
IL-8, 5, 108
immune function, 24
immune response, 36
immune system, 13
immunodeficiency, 60
immunoreactivity, 77, 91
in situ hybridization, 112
in vitro, 63, 67, 68, 77, 79, 81, 88, 90, 93, 104, 106, 108, 111
in vivo, 86, 94
incidence, 1, 53
India, 67, 68
infarction, 26, 43, 106
infection, 7, 26, 42, 46, 49, 51, 52, 60, 79, 97, 112
inflammation, 5, 6, 7, 8, 9, 11, 12, 14, 15, 16, 18, 19, 20, 21, 22, 23, 36, 37, 39, 44, 51, 59, 65, 67, 68, 79, 96, 102, 107, 113
inflammatory cells, 5, 7, 15
inflammatory disease, 79
inflammatory mediators, 12, 13, 28, 57, 64, 68, 69, 104, 107, 111
infliximab, 36

inhibition, 8, 11, 14, 19, 20, 22, 23, 24, 28, 32, 35, 38, 68, 81, 98, 101, 112
inhibitor, 19, 21, 22, 97, 102, 113
initiation, 16
injections, vii, 15, 30, 35, 41, 42, 44, 45, 46, 59, 75, 81, 85, 86, 94, 95, 96, 100
injuries, 59, 80, 95
injury, iv, 1, 2, 3, 4, 5, 6, 8, 9, 18, 21, 32, 37, 38, 43, 45, 52, 69, 73, 82, 99, 102, 113
insomnia, 32, 42
instruments, 71, 94
integrity, 49, 61, 63
interaction, 38, 103
interactions, 106
interference, 30
interferon, 5
interleukins, 5
intervention, vii
intramuscular injection, 31
intravenous drug abusers, 26
intravenously, 15, 51
ion channels, 14, 16, 27
ions, 58
iron, 58
ischemia, 38

J

joint pain, 25, 37, 42, 59, 66, 98, 100
joints, 27, 42, 60, 61, 91
Jordan, 60, 63, 93
juvenile rheumatoid arthritis, 36

K

kinetics, 16
knee arthroplasty, 98
kyphosis, 31, 91

L

laminectomy, 42
latency, 39, 104

lesions, 22
leukotrienes, 15
life expectancy, 73
life satisfaction, 72
ligament, 4, 58, 59, 86, 88
ligand, 10, 13, 24
lipids, 16, 61
liver, 59, 63
liver disease, 63
local anesthetic, vii, 31, 32, 41, 44, 46, 59, 89, 94
localization, 4, 78, 98
locomotor, 82
lymphocytes, 5, 7

M

macrophages, 5, 7, 15, 36
magnetic field, 58, 84
magnetic materials, 58
magnets, 58, 61, 91
maintenance, 101, 102
management, vii, 17, 35, 39, 56, 58, 60, 63, 64, 73, 75, 78, 90, 92, 93, 95, 97, 105, 112
manipulation, 55, 60, 61, 73, 81, 85, 92, 93, 101, 106, 110
mast cells, 5, 7, 13
matrix, 15, 62, 77, 86, 93, 108
matrix metalloproteinase, 15, 77, 86, 93, 108
measures, 3, 63
Medicare, 98
medication, 33, 42, 43, 77, 84, 95, 101, 113
membranes, 19
men, 1, 72, 90
meta-analysis, 62, 78, 105, 113
metabolism, 40, 63, 64, 67, 68
metabolites, 5, 14, 22, 107
metalloproteinase, 15, 64
methylprednisolone, 44, 45
mice, 6, 13, 82, 85, 87, 92, 94, 97, 112
migraine headache, 7
migration, 15, 36, 59
mobility, 57, 62, 66, 68, 72

model, 10, 21, 22, 34, 38, 40, 51, 65, 84, 89, 96, 98, 99, 100, 102, 107, 108, 113
models, 8, 21, 24, 39, 110
mood, 26, 64
morning, 64
morning stiffness, 64
morphine, 3, 6, 8, 10, 24, 25, 33, 34, 39, 41, 43, 47, 48, 65, 77, 78, 83, 90, 99, 101, 105, 108, 109, 111, 112
mortality, 43
mortality rate, 43
motion, 21, 30, 52, 77
motor control, 61, 92
motor neurons, 32
movement, 1, 12, 29, 56, 57, 61
mRNA, 96
multiple sclerosis, 32, 39
muscarinic receptor, 39
muscle relaxant, vii, 34, 35, 44, 68, 89
muscle spasms, 34, 47
muscle strain, 4
muscle strength, 56
muscles, 1, 3, 13, 27, 30, 60, 61, 100

N

narcotic, 26, 34, 103, 110
narcotic analgesics, 103, 110
narcotics, 60
neck injury, 1, 2
necrosis, 36, 90
nerve, vii, 3, 4, 5, 6, 7, 8, 9, 10, 13, 17, 18, 24, 28, 31, 32, 37, 38, 39, 43, 56, 58, 65, 81, 82, 86, 88, 92, 94, 103, 108, 113
nerve fibers, 3, 5, 10, 56
nerve growth factor, 5, 13, 86
Netherlands, 104
neural function, 35
neuralgia, 4, 27, 28, 34, 40, 44, 112
neurokinin, 6, 8, 9, 82, 86, 110
neuronal calcium channels, 100
neurons, 4, 5, 6, 7, 8, 11, 12, 13, 14, 16, 24, 27, 29, 33, 37, 38, 44, 46, 80, 86, 91, 96, 98, 102, 106, 109

neuropathic pain, 8, 11, 26, 28, 32, 33, 34, 37, 38, 39, 40, 41, 43, 46, 47, 77, 79, 80, 82, 83, 85, 90, 91, 96, 97, 99, 106, 107, 110, 111, 112, 113
neuropathy, 33, 34
neuropeptides, 6, 7, 8, 13, 14, 37, 101, 104
neuropharmacology, 104
neurotoxicity, 94
neurotransmission, 47
neurotransmitter, 9
neutrophils, 5
Nigeria, 89
nitric oxide, 5, 7, 11, 12, 62, 64, 65, 92, 93, 107
nitric oxide synthase, 11
nitrogen, 12
NMDA receptors, 11, 33
N-methyl-D-aspartic acid, 112
Nobel Prize, 18
non-steroidal anti-inflammatory drugs, 34, 100, 107
norepinephrine, 12, 34
North America, 105
NSAIDs, 17, 18, 19, 20, 21, 23, 33, 91, 104, 110
nucleus, 93, 102, 107

O

oedema, 82
oil, 59, 63, 68, 96
omega-3, 15, 63, 78, 107
opiates, 39
opioids, 5, 7, 10, 25, 26, 46, 90, 93, 94, 109
oral antibiotic, 52
oral antibiotics, 52
osteoarthritis, 2, 10, 15, 21, 23, 28, 39, 59, 62, 63, 64, 66, 67, 79, 81, 83, 86, 88, 92, 93, 94, 95, 100, 102, 103, 104, 105, 110, 113
osteomyelitis, 2, 26, 49, 50, 51, 52, 78, 81, 85, 86, 87, 88, 93, 97, 100, 106, 108
ovarian cancer, 97

P

pain, vii, 1, 2, 3, 4, 5, 6, 7, 8, 9, 10, 11, 12, 13, 14, 15, 16, 17, 18, 20, 21, 22, 23, 24, 25, 26, 27, 29, 30, 31, 32, 33, 34, 36, 37, 38, 39, 40, 41, 42, 43, 44, 46, 47, 55, 56, 57, 58, 59, 60, 61, 62, 63, 64, 65, 66, 67, 68, 69, 71, 72, 75, 77, 78, 79, 80, 81, 82, 83, 84, 85, 86, 87, 88, 89, 90, 91, 92, 93, 94, 95, 96, 97, 98, 99, 100, 101, 102, 103, 104, 105, 106, 108, 109, 110, 112, 113
pain management, 98
palpation, 57
paralysis, 87
parameters, 31, 84
pathogenesis, 7, 57
pathogens, 49
pathology, 4
pathways, 14, 23, 32, 64, 68, 94, 98, 107
penicillin, 51
peptides, 5, 6, 8, 10, 16, 24
perfusion, 113
periodontal, 67, 106
peripheral neuropathy, 27
phantom limb pain, 33, 112
pharmacology, 86
pharmacotherapy, vii
phenol, 59
phospholipids, 63
phosphorylation, 19
physical activity, 33
physical therapy, vii, 72
physiology, 83
pilot study, 88, 89, 99
placebo, 23, 30, 32, 33, 34, 36, 40, 41, 66, 68, 83, 85, 87, 92, 95, 97, 98, 99, 100, 103, 104, 105, 110, 112
plants, vii, 27, 63, 68
plasma, 7, 110
plasma membrane, 110
platelet aggregation, 22
platelets, 5, 18
polymerase, 84
polymerase chain reaction, 84
polypeptide, 77, 78, 109
polyps, 21
poor, 43, 53, 72
population, 1, 4, 72, 78, 84, 88
potassium, 5, 9, 46
pressure, 12, 56, 57, 61, 85, 90
production, 7, 12, 13, 15, 18, 19, 21, 31, 58, 64, 66, 67, 68, 79, 95, 107, 108, 111
program, 60, 72, 90, 93
proliferation, 64, 90
prophylactic, 50, 51, 103
prophylaxis, 109
prostaglandins, 5, 13, 14, 17, 18, 19, 22, 23, 57, 64, 65, 66, 67, 69, 106
prostate, 103
protein kinase C, 13
protein synthesis, 21
proteins, 18, 36, 61, 62
proteoglycans, 62, 90
proteolytic enzyme, 62, 82
protocol, 58
psoriasis, 36
psoriatic arthritis, 36
purines, 13, 106
pyogenic, 86, 90

Q

quality of life, vii, 25, 43, 56, 59, 71, 72, 81, 101, 105

R

rradiculopathy, 2, 12, 44, 90, 96, 100
range, 1, 11, 26, 30, 52, 56, 58, 61, 79, 82
rash, 22, 37
receptors, 3, 5, 7, 8, 9, 10, 11, 12, 13, 14, 23, 24, 35, 36, 37, 38, 39, 40, 41, 43, 46, 80, 86, 93, 97, 99, 100, 103, 105, 113
recombinant DNA, 37
reconstruction, 86
red blood cells, 45
reflex sympathetic dystrophy, 111
reflexes, 3, 6, 35

regeneration, 59, 91
region, 1, 29, 59
regulation, 9, 11, 16, 23, 82, 93
rehabilitation, 56, 58, 72
rehabilitation program, 72
relaxation, 57, 90
relevance, 97
relief, 3, 25, 27, 40, 41, 42, 43, 44, 46, 47, 57, 60, 61, 68, 69, 72, 75, 86, 92
repair, 16, 59
respiratory, 45, 46
respiratory arrest, 45
responsiveness, 8, 31
rheumatic diseases, 91, 94, 99
rheumatoid arthritis, 7, 15, 21, 28, 36, 37, 39, 57, 58, 60, 63, 66, 67, 68, 78, 85, 90, 96, 112
rhizome, 95
risk, 21, 26, 43, 60, 104
RNA, 7, 64, 78
RNA processing, 78

S

safety, 79, 91, 100
sciatica, 37, 44, 89
scores, 21, 41, 56, 71, 72, 91
sedative, 32, 68
self-regulation, 93
sensation, 1, 6, 11, 16, 27, 28, 82, 108
sensing, 16, 111
sensitivity, 3, 7, 11, 15, 52, 57, 78
sensitization, 4, 5, 12, 14, 18, 24, 80, 83, 89
septic arthritis, 88
septic discitis, 51
serotonin, 5, 7, 19, 23, 55, 57, 80, 105
serum, 12, 50, 97
severity, 3, 25, 29
sexual behavior, 86
shoulders, 58, 72
sickle cell, 96
side effects, 14, 26, 41, 46, 105
signal transduction, 18
signals, 14, 15, 107
signs, 52, 68

skeletal muscle, 32, 56, 107
skin, 7, 22, 39, 43, 58, 89, 103, 108
smooth muscle, 15
social class, 78
sodium, 16, 22, 34, 80, 87, 94, 95
soybean, 88
space, 26, 42, 49, 51, 61, 112
spasticity, 32, 35, 43, 47, 77, 110
species, 12, 49, 52
spectrum, 52, 112
spinal anesthesia, 53
spinal cord, 5, 6, 7, 8, 9, 11, 26, 33, 34, 35, 37, 38, 39, 43, 44, 45, 46, 47, 52, 79, 91, 93, 96, 98, 100, 101, 103, 104, 106, 108, 110, 113
spinal cord injury, 34, 37, 39, 44, 45, 47, 79, 93, 96, 98, 106, 108, 110
spinal fusion, 86
spinal stenosis, 44
spine, 1, 2, 25, 26, 36, 42, 43, 45, 46, 49, 51, 52, 66, 72, 81, 82, 92, 97, 104, 106, 110, 111, 113
spore, 29
sprains, 3, 4, 27, 59
staphylococci, 50, 83, 95
stenosis, 42, 60
steroids, vii, 42, 44, 60, 64, 67, 96
stimulus, 59, 80, 82
stomach, 18, 66
strabismus, 30
strain, 2, 32, 40, 44
strategies, 72, 75
strength, 25, 58, 65, 67, 79
streptococci, 50
stress, 37, 72
subgroups, 106, 111
substance use, 26
suppression, 28, 29, 37, 43, 68, 112
sympathetic nervous system, 12, 13
symptom, 4, 40
symptoms, 29, 37, 40, 42, 59, 63, 64, 65, 112
synaptic transmission, 113
syndrome, 2, 25, 28, 30, 34, 37, 42, 45, 46, 47, 56, 81, 88, 95, 102, 108

Index

synergistic effect, 36
synovial fluid, 21, 28, 50, 97, 106
synovial membrane, 99
synovial tissue, 105
synovitis, 8, 15, 42, 90
synthesis, 19, 22, 23, 44, 61, 62, 64, 68, 69, 86, 90, 98, 108

T

T cell, 68, 99
targets, 22, 75
teicoplanin, 51
temperature, 16, 28, 37
tendon, 21, 58, 59, 77, 90
tension, 32, 34, 56
tension headache, 32, 34
terminals, 10, 16, 18, 24, 35
thalamus, 39, 93
therapeutic agents, 81
therapists, 107
therapy, 25, 26, 30, 31, 34, 36, 41, 51, 52, 55, 57, 58, 59, 62, 65, 67, 72, 77, 78, 84, 89, 91, 92, 93, 94, 95, 105, 106
threshold, 6, 14, 16, 23, 28, 57, 61, 88, 91, 92, 93
thresholds, 30, 41, 85, 101
thromboxanes, 14
tissue, 3, 4, 5, 7, 8, 12, 15, 16, 21, 27, 49, 52, 58, 59, 86, 95, 103, 108
TNF, vii, 5, 36, 62, 64, 65, 102, 107, 111
TNF-alpha, 62, 65, 102, 107, 111
tonic, 30, 38
torsion, 30
toxin, 28, 29, 30, 31, 35, 73, 81, 82, 84, 88, 91, 94, 102, 104, 109, 113
training, 60, 79, 93
transformation, 107
transforming growth factor, 15
transmission, 6, 11, 12, 14, 16, 19, 38, 46, 94
transport, 31, 81, 86

trapezius, 13, 44
trauma, 4, 18, 53, 57
trial, 21, 32, 33, 78, 79, 81, 83, 85, 88, 89, 92, 94, 97, 101, 102, 105, 109, 112
tricyclic antidepressant, 35, 41
tricyclic antidepressants, 35
trigeminal neuralgia, 28, 34
triggers, 15
tuberculosis, 84
tumor, vii, 5, 36, 69, 97, 113
tumor necrosis factor, vii, 5, 36, 97, 113

U

ultrasound, 72, 103
United States, 29, 37, 42, 44, 62, 64
uric acid, 69

V

vancomycin, 50, 51, 84
vasoactive intestinal peptide, 5, 6
vasoconstriction, 31
vasodilator, 7, 114
vasomotor, 28
vegetables, 68
venlafaxine, 80
ventricle, 113
vertebral artery, 42

W

weakness, 27, 31, 59
women, 1, 72, 90

Z

zinc, 105